Bulimia Is A
Dental Disease

Bulimia Is A Dental Disease

Brian McKay, DDS

To order additional copies of this book, contact:
Xlibris Corporation
1-888-795-4274
www.Xlibris.com
Orders@Xlibris.com
40306

CONTENTS

A MESSAGE FROM DR. GREGORY L. JANTZ, PHD, CEDS 9

FOREWORD 13

ACKNOWLEDGMENTS 15

INTRODUCTION 17

CHAPTER 1: A STANDARD OF CARE ISSUE 21

CHAPTER 2: BULIMIA: A SEARCH FOR MEANING 29

CHAPTER 3: BODY AND SOUL: THE PHYSICAL
             AND PSYCHOLOGICAL IMPACT OF BULIMIA 50

CHAPTER 4: BULIMIA IS A DENTAL DISEASE 68

CHAPTER 5: STEP 1: FACE-TO-FACE WITH BULIMIA 76

CHAPTER 6: STEP 2: LET TREATMENT BEGIN! 100

CHAPTER 7: STEP 3: LEARNING TO SMILE AGAIN 119

CHAPTER 8: STEP 4: A WORK IN PROGRESS 130

CHAPTER 9: THE RECOVERY CHEST 148

CHAPTER 10: QUESTIONS AND ANSWERS 170

APPENDIX 183

SUGGESTED READING LIST 188

This book is dedicated to the memory of my sainted mother, Kathleen Tierney McKay. She taught her children there was no limit to the amount of love to share with those in need. To "love more, judge less". And that there is always a place at the dinner table for one more . . . .

A Message from
Dr. Gregory L. Jantz, PhD, CEDS

I've been working with eating disorders for practically all of my adult life. Over that time, I've come into contact with many healthcare professionals. Some have shown little patience with the complexities of an eating disorder, preferring to deal with the disorder through a "here's a pill—just don't do it anymore" approach. My personal frustration at this approach is nothing compared to the despair of the person suffering from the eating disorder. You can imagine, then, my appreciation of and delight in the insights, passion and commitment of Dr. Brian McKay.

Here is a dental professional with a rare knowledge and understanding of the many faces of an eating disorder. This book is titled "Bulimia is a Dental Disease" but Dr. McKay shows he is also well versed in anorexia and purging disorder. His presentation is non-judgmental, springing from a heart of compassion and a professional commitment to bring hope and restoration. This is not a dry, clinical recitation of facts. Rather, it is an interactive read, with invaluable suggestions and guidelines. You'll also hear—in their own words—from patients Dr. McKay has worked with over the years, who are today experiencing healing from their eating disorder.

For those with eating disorders, a visit to the dentist can represent a cry for help, with damage to the teeth as merely the tip of the iceberg. As such, dentists are on the front lines of detection and in a unique position to present truth to their patients. This book is about truth telling, springing from Dr. McKay's passion to understand bulimia and associated eating disorders from a professional point of view, in order to offer help to you on a personal level. Reading between the lines of this comprehensive presentation, you can feel Dr. McKay's outrage at the devastation wrought by an eating disorder, not only the dental damage but also the physical, psychological and spiritual damage.

Make no mistake, this book was written just for you. If you are suffering from an eating disorder, Dr. McKay wants you to know there is hope and restoration. If you are concerned about a loved one, this book offers an excellent overview of eating disorders and treatment options, as well as thoughtful suggestions on how—and how not—to express your care and concern. If you are a dental professional—or any healthcare professional, for that matter—this book can rekindle the fire of advocacy for those afflicted with such a devastating disease.

For those suffering from an eating disorder, recovery has several milestones. Even after the purging behavior has stopped, recovery continues, as the person heals and moves toward reclaiming a "normal" life. But how normal is it not to smile? How normal is it to avoid opening your mouth or engaging in conversation out of shame for the condition of your teeth? That shame taps into the shame and negativity of the eating disorder. Dr. McKay knows this and has seen first-hand how a smile releases shame. By reclaiming a smile, a person can reclaim a return to health and normalcy. When they look in the mirror, they see their present and future smiling back at them, not a grim reminder of the past.

As I said earlier, it's rare to find someone as committed to restoration as Dr. McKay. His dedication to providing answers and hope is so encompassing, he felt compelled to write it down in this book. I can only hope that your desire to know more, to know healing, is compelling enough for you to read it. I have; more, I've lived it over the past several years through my association with Dr. McKay and his amazing staff of dedicated, caring professionals.

Many people in the midst of an eating disorder feel they're all alone, that no one else cares. That's not true. I care and so does Dr. McKay. Read this book and let it speak to your heart. You will hear many voices clambering for your attention where an eating disorder is concerned. Let Dr. McKay's clear message of hope and restoration inspire you to work for healing and recovery, whether you are a sufferer yourself, or know of someone suffering, or work in the dental or medical field. There are too few voices like Dr. McKay's speaking out in our world; when one speaks, we all need to listen.

With sincere gratitude,
Dr. Gregory L. Jantz, PhD, CEDS

FOREWORD

I've known Dr. Brian McKay for over a dozen years. We studied together in the very early days of the aesthetic dental revolution that changed the way reconstructive dentistry is delivered. As we advanced in our studies, we both became teachers and helped thousands of dentists fulfill their hopes and dreams to become world-class clinicians.

He is an excellent dental practitioner, on the cutting edge of aesthetic dentistry—caring and concerned for his patients and their overall health. That's why it's no surprise to see that Brian has authored a book about bulimia and the devastation it brings not just to the mouth and its structures but to the patients and their families.

Extensively researched and written in an easy-to-understand way, Brian lays out what bulimia is, how it attacks the teeth and soft tissues of the mouth and what we should, as dentists, be doing about it. I was astounded to learn that dentists first diagnose 26 percent of bulimic cases.

Brian is challenging clinicians, and dentistry as a whole, with this book. He is saying, "We are on the front line when it comes to recognizing the symptoms and participating in the solution." It is time to wake up. It is time to step up and it is time to take responsibility. That is Brian's message to the dental professional.

Yes, we can restore the mouth and reverse the damage done but are we treating the whole patient? Do we not have an obligation to refer the individual in our dental chair to the proper therapists, psychologists and treatment professionals to complete her restoration? Dr. McKay suggests that we do have that obligation. He shows us how to approach a patient with empathy and understanding. He relates his own successful approach to the difficult and sometimes impossible task of reaching out in a non-judgmental way to comfort the patient and guide them toward treatment of their disease.

Not every bulimic patient is ready to resolve his or her issues and stop purging. Bulimia is a complex and insidious disease that strikes the most vulnerable at their weakest point. It creates controversy at every meal, every snack, every drink and every day. The struggle is long, hard and full of pitfalls. It isn't about food as much as it is about expectations and image and personal choices we cannot begin to understand.

Reading this book caused me to reflect on the pain, the hopelessness and difficulty bulimics and their families face daily. I know as a clinician that I can restore their mouth but it is more than that. Their whole life has to be restored. They have to learn how to live with food and understand the positives that life has to offer. This book shows us how to start the process.

I wish my friend well with this book and I urge all dental practitioners to read it. I encourage them to pass it on to others in the field and to give it to patients whom they perceive to be suffering with an eating disorder. I know I will.

David Hornbrook, DDS, FAACD
Executive Director, Hornbrook Group Center for Dental Studies
www.hornbrookgroup.com
San Diego, CA

ACKNOWLEDGMENTS

Writing this book was not an easy task. There are many people who influenced me, guided me and taught me along the way. The book would not have been possible without their kindness, their patience and their hard work. I wish to thank the following people for their efforts in helping me get to the place where this book could be completed:

Greg Jantz, Ph.D—pioneer, visionary, friend, mentor and leader in the Eating Disorder community.

Laura Minor, MSW-C, CDP—hard working, dedicated and selfless Eating Disorder specialist.

Jillianne S.—a struggling soul ravaged by bulimia. We miss her.

Diane F.—someone who has overcome her Eating Disorder and become a close friend as well as my patient.

Laura B.—a woman whom I admire both for her tenacity and her kindness.

Aimee F.—she is fighting the good fight and she has me in her corner.

Megan. R.—who touched my heart like no other.

David Hornbrook, DDS, FAACD—a friend and colleague, a teacher, lecturer, writer and genius.

Tanya Goodman—she is tenacious, a tireless researcher and ED advocate and has been a vital player in this program. Her ability to relate as an ED partner has fostered our growth in this field.

Mike Faber—for over 25 years he has counseled and kept me pointed in the right direction. We have a great partnership. He was essential in bringing this book out from the get-go.

Deborah Mitchell—I thank her for her research and editorial assistance
    with this book. Thank you so much Debbie.
And, Tim, Kelli and Scott. My children who mean the world to me.

                                        Brian McKay, DDS
                                        Seattle, WA

INTRODUCTION

In the process of writing this book people would ask me not about the content of the book but the intent of the book. So, I thought I'd take a moment and tell you what this book is about and what it isn't.

As the first book dedicated to pointing out the absolute link between bulimia and a specific dental condition brought on by bulimia there is a lot to cover. You'll learn how a dentist knows a patient is bulimic just by looking in the patient's mouth. We'll meet some courageous women and men who share their stories about eating disorders. I am most honored that they have shared their stories with me and with you.

This is not another bulimia book although we discuss bulimia throughout. This is not a medical science book although medical science is shared with the reader. This book is not a psychological treatise although psychology and various psychological methods of treatment are presented. This is not a dental book either, although dentists play a significant role in this book and the strong link between bulimia and dentistry is defined and explored. This book is more than that.

This book supports a vision I have for it and for all people who suffer from bulimia. Whether you have yet faced your disease and are on the road to conquering it or your eating disorder still has you in it's grasp—my message is clear. You don't have to worry and wait until you are losing or have lost your teeth. Get to a dentist now. Tell the dentist of your concerns, show your teeth and smile and then ask for help. We will know what to do. We can repair your smile; we can participate in your healing. We can help restore your self-esteem and help build your confidence.

My message to dentists is to wake up! There is a world of suffering, tormented young women and men in need of your training and tender, loving care. If dentists are discovering 26-28% of all bulimia either that number is too low or too high. In my opinion, it's too low. Dentists everywhere must become proactive in recognizing, diagnosing and treating the bulimic dental patient. And every bulimic patient should be under a dentist's care.

This book is the foundation for that. You will learn about how bulimia and dentistry are linked. You will discover what to look for if you are a bulimic, the parent of a bulimic or you are one of the professionals working in the eating disorder field. A field, I might add, that is filled with dedicated, heart-felt care and caring from strong people.

The problem is simply overwhelming. Billions are spent annually driving the image of an emaciated standard of beauty and success that just isn't true. This image presents itself very early in the life of a bulimic and intertwines with a desire to achieve, twisting that desire into a compulsion that is easy to hide, justify and ultimately live with until it is appears to be too late. That is how this disease works. It changes the thinking patterns of its victims until those twisted patterns drive the life of the victim into misery.

Bingeing and purging are the names we use to describe what is really a complex condition that involves so much more than bingeing and purging. For example, the purging ruins teeth over time by stripping the enamel and attacking the teeth with stomach acid. You'll learn why brushing right after purging is a bad thing.

The proceeds from this book will go to the **SMILE WITHIN FOUNDATION**. Started to ensure the achievement of the original goal—to shine a light on the connection between bulimia and dentistry and to show that bulimia nervosa is attacking teeth thus creating a disease environment that, if left unchecked, may result in loss of all the victim's teeth. The purpose of the foundation is twofold: to educate dental professionals about Eating Disorders including how to approach communication and treatment of bulimics and secondly to provide underwriting for the successful dental restoration of deserving yet financially strapped bulimia and purging disorder victims.

My hope is that this book will be the book that dentists everywhere give to their eating disorder patients. It is my further hope that Eating

Disorder professionals will read it and understand that dentists everywhere are their allies and should be considered as part of their support team in treating these devastating conditions.

When I graduated from dental school in 1980, it never occurred to me that one day, more than twenty-five years later, I would be writing a book about bulimia. Why would a dentist write about bulimia? Sure, I had *heard* about bulimia in dental school. It was presented, as so many other dental and medical conditions were, in terms of how it manifested in the *body*. Thus, the eating disorder known as bulimia nervosa was reduced to (and I am over-simplifying it here) a set of signs and symptoms: erosion of the enamel of the teeth (primarily the backs of the front teeth), as well as inflamed parotid glands, gingivitis, and facial pain, among others. It was portrayed not as a disease that affects the emotional, physical, social, and spiritual essence of a human being, but as a complex of physical manifestations that could be treated according to standardized dental procedures and techniques. And to the best of my recollection, I don't recall any of the professors advising us to discuss our suspicions with the patients. We were, after all, *dental* students, not students of psychiatry or endocrinology or internal medicine.

Which brings me to the title of this book. I know bulimia is not only a dental disease. Indeed, bulimia is a complex, multifaceted, psychological disorder that affects females primarily (at least 10 percent of eating disorder victims are male and the number is growing) and which has a profound effect on the body, mind, and soul of those who suffer with it. But for bulimics and their families and friends, the fact that this disease, which bulimics typically can hide from their spouses, family members, friends, and the world so well, announces itself to the world *through the mouth* so to speak; the fact that dentists are in a unique position, as health-care professionals, to detect the disease, even in its early stages, well before other medical practitioners can or do (if indeed they do), prompts me to refer to bulimia as a dental disease.

And I will continue to do so because I want to get your attention, just like Megan and Diane and Laura and Abigail and Mariah and Aimee and many others with bulimia got mine when they walked into my office and I saw the heart-breaking results of this insidious disease—the decayed, crumbling, fractured teeth, the traumatized gums and mucus membranes, and the swollen salivary glands. I want your attention, whether you have bulimia or you love or care about someone who does; whether you're a partner, parent, best friend; an educator, a physician, a therapist, or a dentist. I want your attention because bulimia is a serious, life-threatening, physically, emotionally, and spiritually devastating disease that impacts the lives of a millions of females and males, mostly young but increasingly among older people, in the United States. Some of these individuals are as young as six years of age. Many others have been living with the disease and all the turmoil—the shame, low self-esteem, embarrassment, guilt—that goes along with it for decades.

You—they—deserve and need information, support, understanding, and treatment. You need to know that all of these things are available to you, right here and now. You need to know that many former bulimics have broken free of the bonds of bulimia, turned the corner, and embraced their health, their smile, and their lives. I know because I am involved in some of those lives, in the breaking free, in helping restore the smile and self-confidence. I work closely with psychologist and eating disorder specialist Gregory L. Jantz, PhD, founder and director of The Center for Counseling and Health Resources, Inc., in Edmonds, Washington, and with specialists and patients associated with other programs.

In this book you will, I hope, learn things that will erase your fears and misconceptions about the disease, and then use the resources offered—be they facts, checklists, resource materials, or the words of hope and inspiration from the many stories shared within these pages—to restore your life or that of a loved one. In some places in this book you have the opportunity to not only read about how someone won her battle against this disease, but hear the story as well: I have included links to my website where you can listen to testimonials from recovering and recovered bulimics as well as see before-and-after photos of some of the cosmetic dentistry done on these individuals.

I love what I do: every day I have an opportunity to change people's lives through restorative cosmetic dentistry. But the most gratifying and humbling part of my work is when I can help people who are struggling with bulimia get the help they want and need and play a role in restoring and recreating their smiles—smiles that light up their entire being and touch me every time. To protect privacy, I've changed some of the names in this book but none of the stories.

CHAPTER 1

A STANDARD OF CARE ISSUE

Her name was Megan. She was 26 years old when we met. She weighed a mere 71 lbs. at that time. She had been both anorexic and bulimic since the age of 12. Her life was tragic. She lived in a waking nightmare 24/365. Bingeing and purging consumed her when she wasn't starving herself. The diseases controlled every action, every thought, every dream and every waking moment. She was imprisoned by the stark reality of trying to live with a terrible eating disorder. It had begun to consume the very tissues of her body. Bone began to resorb, her teeth became loose and fell out as the bone around them shrunk and became brittle. Her body was starved for nutrients as she vomited throughout the early morning hours to rid herself of what little food she retained. She was in the throes of full-blown bulimia and anorexia. At 26, most people still have all 32 teeth but Megan had only 12 when I met her—six upper and six lower. Her teeth and gums reminded me of someone in their 70's, someone who had experienced a lifetime of neglect.

Her existence revolved around sleeping a very troubled sleep during the day and consuming massive amounts of food at night to fuel her purging activity. Her daily routine was to lie in bed throughout the day, not eating, restless, tossing and turning too exhausted to find that deep, comforting sleep we all need to feel better. Megan never felt better during those times.

She only slept a total of two or three hours a day before the disease would force her to stumble her way into the kitchen, usually between 11pm and midnight every night long after her mother and siblings would tuck themselves in. For Megan, the night was a blur of cooking, eating and finally purging before throwing herself into bed again desperately in need of rest and rejuvenation but the starving, tossing and turning would start all over night after night, day after day.

"I usually eat about 10 lbs. of potatoes most nights because you can cook them so many ways. I go through about a dozen eggs, two or three sticks of butter, a half-gallon of milk, whole boxes of cookies and crackers. Often, I would eat an entire watermelon, seeds, rind—everything but the skin, because it was easy to purge. My mother stopped bringing cakes and boxes of doughnuts into the house because by morning they would be all gone. Down the toilet every night," she said. "I would starve myself during the day. I had no energy to do anything. I don't even remember what it feels like to be healthy," she told me.

Megan, like most eating disorder victims, struggled alone and in secret until the physical toll on her body became too much for her to handle on her own. She told her family of her secret after passing out from sheer hunger. She was in both emotional and physical distress. She had reached a crisis point. At first, the family was confused, in denial almost and did not know what to do. After getting over the shock and reading up on these diseases, they sought treatment for her, first in an outpatient-counseling program. Sadly, that did not work.

Megan, similar to many others with the same disorder, relapsed into the living nightmare once again. Bingeing and purging every night. It became too much to look at herself in the mirror. The anorexia worked on her mind and convinced her she did not need to gain any weight but she did express a desire to get better, knowing it would help her and her family in the long run. Then a series of both in-patient and outpatient treatment centers near her home tried to work with her. Unfortunately, she was unable to turn the corner on her health and they failed. Upon completion of the formal treatment, she was returned to home and soon resumed the same pattern as before. Only now, she was a ghost of her former self. She started to lose even more body weight and even more teeth. That is when she came to the attention of the team of experts who reached out to her on all possible levels. That is when she finally started to make some progress. It also was where she came face to face with the underlying reasons for her condition. She began to open up about the sexual abuse that had triggered everything. But her physical condition demanded that she received immediate dental treatment. She was in acute pain when I learned about her.

My good friend and professional colleague, Dr. Greg Jantz from The Center for Counseling and Health Resources in Edmonds, Washington contacted me about treating Megan's dental problems. Dr. Jantz and I had had frank discussions about how bulimia attacked the mouth and how carefully one had to approach these fragile victims in order to successfully treat them. She was suffering with a very loose front tooth that was causing her unrelenting pain and she needed to see a dentist immediately. We obliged and arranged to see Megan as soon as possible. When she arrived two things struck me right away. First, she was in dire need of full mouth reconstruction not just emergency care. Her mouth was in bad shape. It wasn't just the loose tooth in the front. There were many missing teeth, severe gum disease, bone loss and a few abscesses. Her salivary glands were swollen and red. Bulimia had ravaged her mouth almost to the point of total loss.

Secondly, this waif of a woman had volumes of character and strength deep within her that were untapped. Her spirit shone through the trauma she was experiencing as she looked me right in the eye and said, "I want to get better I want you to help me." My heart broke into a thousand million pieces. Her very presence impressed my entire office staff and me. She was a fighter and had been fighting alone for so long. It touched me far beyond my professional veneer and I was moved emotionally. In my entire career of over 20 years as a dentist, that had never happened before. I knew she was special. I knew I had to help her. My staff felt exactly the same way and came to me after her first visit and told me "whatever it takes, let's make this girl whole again."

Previous dentists had treated her mouth by extracting teeth and not much else. Had they failed to recognize the severity of her condition? Had they failed to see the whole person sitting in their dental chair? Was she viewed as just a mouth with a person attached? Why hadn't previous dentists talked to her in a non-judgmental way? Why hadn't they gone the extra mile and recognized what a valuable human being Megan was?

I had treated many bulimics in my office before Megan. Most had "turned the corner" and were well along the way toward recovery. Their teeth were usually the last thing they addressed in their treatment many telling me that their teeth and smile reminded them of that time in their lives when they were not in control. They were ashamed to smile. This patient, however, was still in the throes of the disease and needed immediate care.

I approach them all in a very non-judgmental way. Too many dentists and their staffs assume a parental role in treating their patients scolding them to brush and floss better. It has been years since I did that with my patients. I found that it just doesn't work. People feel bad enough about their teeth. Why should I, or my staff wag their finger and admonish the patient about their oral hygiene and the condition of their mouth? It is what it is. And it is our responsibility to fix it.

Too often, there is a "back office buzz" about patients and their personal lives. That does not occur in my practice. The success rate with patients soared when I stopped being their parent and became their practitioner. I want to restore their smiles not be their parent. With bulimics and anorexics it is the same only much more intense. They will not return to your practice if you make them feel worse than they already do. It's as simple as that.

Almost any dentist with advanced cosmetic training is equipped to handle the dental needs of an eating disorder victim but I am saddened by their inability to deal with the whole person. The reason seems to be that a lot of dentists publicly judge their patient. They are not yet aware of the non-judgmental approach needed to successfully treat and complete the treatment of their patients, let alone someone dealing with a challenge much larger than dental.

Dentists must learn how to become successful in talking to their patients. Most dentists can do a decent diagnosis and relate their findings to the patient. But then they lapse into the parental role. I am told all the time by dentists whom I taught or mentored, "Well, you can do that because of who you are." My response is that it is a learned behavior. "How well could you drill a tooth before dental school," I ask. The answer is "not very well". That leads me to ask why they think they cannot learn how to relate to people. It is a learned skill just like drilling teeth. It takes practice, commitment and dedication—just like the rest of dentistry.

Once the dentist learns to meet people "where they live", once they learn about who their patient is and what motivates them, then they also learn that the patient will accept treatment. I have to credit one of my mentors for helping me to grow into this role. Tony Robbins, the noted author and lecturer, taught me the Platinum Rule. It is stronger than the Golden Rule, which states, "Treat others as you would like to be treated." While the Platinum Rule is "Treat others as they would like to be treated." Another mentor, Walter Hailey of Dental Boot Kamp and Crown Council fame told me, "The more you know about your patient, the more they think you know about dentistry." That is the essence of relationship building with patients and the key to working successfully with bulimics and other eating disorder patients. Treating bulimics was the natural next step in my development, in my professional odyssey from dental student to wanting to be all things to all patients to realizing that I only wanted to treat people who were ready to take the next step in their own personal development. A bulimic's goal is to just be normal again. As I said, they usually have their teeth restored near the end of or after the end of their clinical recovery. Invariably they will all say the same thing to me:

"This allows me to be whole again. To smile to myself again" I am just restoring their teeth, but to them I am giving them their life back. I am releasing the smile within.

My staff mobilized quickly and we spiritually gathered around Megan in order to provide her a level of treatment that she had never received before. To resolve the immediate issue of the loose front tooth there was no other option but to remove it.

We realized that this would be a further traumatic event for her so we took some time to explain that it was not the end but the beginning of her dental recovery. By removing the front tooth we would relieve the pain immediately and dramatically. She was frightened. She had lost teeth before and hadn't had them replaced. It had always been a financial issue. To save a tooth took a lot more money than to remove it. Her financial resources were tapped out. She could not work. She lived at home. Her mother was a single mom with additional children at home and life was a struggle. We weren't looking for compensation. Dr. Jantz and I decided very early that we would provide all possible care for Megan at no cost whatsoever to her and her family. It was the least we could do. We were trying to save a life. Money was not important in this case. Megan had moved into Dr. Jantz's facility where she could get the highest level of counseling and treatment and my team adopted her for the duration of her care. We even went on television along with Megan to share her story and to motivate our community.

We took the time to explain to Megan that the tooth removal was necessary and we would provide her with a temporary replacement while we designed a new smile for her. It was a complicated case. She would need expert care from a gum specialist to neutralize the gum disease before we could begin the process of restoring her smile. In the meantime, we removed not one but two of her front teeth as we discovered both were infected. We designed a temporary acrylic appliance that would allow her to smile and feel good about herself while the tissue healed. The plan called for aggressive gum treatment and a combination of general and cosmetic dentistry. She would have dental implants placed and teeth would be saved with root canals and crowns. Eventually she would have a completely new smile, 28 teeth to properly eat with and smile into the mirror with.

Tragically, before the work could be completed Megan suffered a major setback and had to return to her home in another state. This often happens with active bulimics as they struggle to keep their heads above water. Neither Dr. Jantz nor I have heard from her since. Phones have been disconnected, mail has been returned and she seems to have disappeared. We hope she is alive. We hope she has sought treatment and counseling. We hope she is eating normally again but we cannot be sure. We have been honored to know her and to experience her spirit. We wish her every success but the old adage applies—you can lead a horse to water but you cannot make the horse drink.

Both Dr. Jantz and I believe that dentistry for bulimics should be included in the Standard of Care. This may appear to be a radical concept when contemplated for the first time. However there is not an eating disorder treatment specialist practicing today that does not realize that bulimia wrecks the teeth and mouth of bulimics and that restoration improves their self-esteem, makes them feel whole again and finally helps to put their disease behind them. A new smile is a wondrous thing not only to behold but also to own. On a practical level, there needs to be a meeting of the minds between the eating disorder treatment specialist world and the dental world. By integrating the two fields, teams can be formed that treat the entire person. From there a standard of care will emerge and a safety net will form around these patients in which all of their fears can be put to rest and we can successfully treat the mind and the body completely and with amazing results.

There are tens of thousands of Megans out there and thousands of Michaels too. Each is suffering in his or her own way with this terrible disease. Children as young as 9 years of age are turning up at treatment centers like Dr. Jantz's in Edmonds, Washington. How does this happen? Is it an indictment of our society? Is it a symptom of something much larger at work? This book examines what bulimia and purging disorders are and illustrates the uncertainty of a professional community that is struggling to catch up with it. It also puts things into perspective for the dental professional. My hope is to enlighten many and motivate a few to take the next step. Learn how to talk to these fragile personalities. Treat them as whole human beings and follow up on their care. It takes years for them to complete their treatment and address the underlying issues that spark the disorder. I am sounding the clarion call to my fellow dentists to become aware, to become advocates of change and to work hand in hand with eating disorder clinics and professionals in turning this preventable situation around. You just need to see the smile within emerge to be convinced that you are a vital part of the success equation for eating disorder victims.

For everyone who seeks treatment there are thousands who do not. What happens to bulimics who do not turn the corner on their disease? Few die from bulimia, however many do die from anorexia—the most fatal of all mental illnesses. Their organs shut down and they pass a point of no return. Anorexia is the only mental disease that people suffer physical death from—as much as 15% to 20% of anorexics die from it including Terri Shiavo, Karen Carpenter, Audrey Hepburn and Margaux Hemingway. Bulimics, those who do not succeed in growing past their disease usually stop purging at some point but keep devouring massive amounts of food. They are not recovered and because they are not rid of the underlying problems that drove them to eat excessively in the first place, they become morbidly obese. Obesity may kill them, may give them a heart attack, stroke or diabetes or another weight related condition. This is what Princess Diana said about her own suffering, "I had bulimia for a number of years. And that's like a secret disease. You inflict it upon yourself because your self-esteem is at low ebb, and you don't think you're worthy or valuable. You fill your stomach up four or five times a day—some do it more—and it gives you a feeling of comfort. It's like having a pair of arms around you, but it's temporary. Then you're disgusted at the bloatedness of your stomach, and you bring it all up again. It's a repetitive pattern, which is very destructive to yourself."

BOTTOM LINE

You don't have to be famous to have an eating disorder. This is a mental disorder that triggers eating or starving—both are extremely damaging and both go hand in hand with each other. Both are symptoms of much larger issues and problems. This book will explain exactly how bulimia ravages the psyche as well as the teeth and mouth. It explains how to talk to an eating disorder patient as well as sharing the stories of many eating disorder victims. Perhaps one will touch you in the same way I was touched by Megan. Perhaps you will find it in yourself to understand a little bit more about eating disorders and the damage that they cause.

I urge dentists and eating disorder professionals to contact me at the email address included in this book to learn more about how they can identify, talk to and treat bulimics and purgers. Perhaps together we can make a difference. Perhaps together we make a change. Perhaps together we can release the smile within.

CHAPTER 2

BULIMIA: A SEARCH FOR MEANING

"I've been bulimic for six years, and my husband doesn't even know it," says Rhonda, a twenty-four-year-old research assistant. "If I tell him, I'm afraid he'll think I'm horrible and disgusting and that he'll leave me. But I don't know how much longer I can hide it. We want to have a family, but I don't know if I can go through a pregnancy and keep bingeing and purging. I'm so afraid."

"I know I have a problem with food. I know I'm bulimic, and have been since I was thirteen." Mona's voice drops to a whisper. "But I can't tell anyone. Every time I throw up I feel so ashamed. I hate myself. I know it's a disgusting habit and that I could die, but I can't stop."

"I'm not really bulimic, because I looked up the definition," says thirty-year-old Tanya defiantly. "And I don't gorge or binge on lots of food like bulimics do. But I do throw up most of what I eat. So does my best friend. I heard that what we do is called purging disorder, and I know that it's ruining my teeth and probably my throat and stomach. I'll have to stop some day, but right now I can't. Sometimes I feel like I want to die."

"I starting throwing up after I ate because I needed to meet weight for the wrestling team," explains seventeen-year-old Roger. "It seemed like the perfect solution: I could eat all I wanted and then just get rid of it. It worked great. But now I can't stop, even though I don't feel so good."

"I've been fighting bulimia for more than twenty years," says Candace, who is now forty-five. "I've seen several therapists for depression, but none of them ever knew I was bulimic. I couldn't tell them, and they never guessed. I get better for a while, and then go back to bingeing and purging several times a day for months. It's been a roller coaster ride, and I don't see it ever ending."

The voices of bulimics resonate with so many raw emotions: despair, self-hatred, fear, disgust, denial, hopelessness, and confusion. Yet to their family and friends and the rest of the world, the face that bulimics typically present tells a different story: they are our sisters, our daughters, our mothers, our best friends, our sons, our neighbors, and our cousins. Generally they tend to be conscientious, perfectionists, sensitive, kind, caring, hard-working, intelligent women and men, who just so happen to be struggling with emotional issues expressed through destructive bulimic behavior.

That behavior generally sets the definition of the disease: an eating disorder characterized by out-of-control eating (bingeing) followed by one or more types of purging activities (self-induced vomiting being the most common approach), which provides the individual with temporary relief from emotional turmoil and/or depression. Yet no definition can begin to express the emotional, mental, physical, and spiritual pain associated with this disease, nor clears up the confusion and fear many people feel when they hear the word "bulimia."

Every day, more and more young girls and boys join the ranks of those who live with this eating disorder. Millions of young people, adolescents, and people in their prime are literally flushing their lives down the toilet, and the number is growing at record rates. The time for the fear, confusion, and denial to end is long past due. So let's begin now.

In this chapter we begin to peel away the layers of bulimia so you can begin to understand this disorder, both by seeing it through the eyes of individuals who have the disease and/or who are in recovery and through information from the scientific literature. We also talk about purging disorder (PD), a clinical condition separate from bulimia in which individuals frequently purge but do not binge. Recent research suggests that PD may be more common than anorexia and bulimia combined. Given that purging is the behavior that has serious medical consequences, you need to understand this condition as well, as it may be even more difficult to detect than bulimia.

LAYING THE FOUNDATION

Before I launch into an exploration of bulimia, I think it's important to highlight two critical points.

- Bulimia, and indeed all eating disorders and their variations, are complex conditions for which there are many gray areas and no clearly drawn lines. Although the book *Diagnostic and Statistical Manual of Mental Disorders IV* (**the** authority to which medical professionals and others turn for the criteria for mental disorders) lists the established criteria and definitions for different eating disorders, in real life people don't follow those "rules." People who have eating disorders often cross the lines and engage in more than one type of so-called "disordered eating" activity. For example, many bulimics will occasionally severely restrict their food intake, which is characteristic of anorexia, the more common of the two eating disorders. Conversely, some anorexics engage in bingeing and/or purging, either occasionally or infrequently. Self-induced vomiting is the main form of purging used by bulimics, although some exercise excessively in an attempt to work off any calories they have consumed. People with anorexia, however, also engage in such obsessive exercise activities. Therefore, I will—with the help of dozens of courageous people who have or who are in recovery from bulimia—attempt to present bulimia in all its shades, from white to black and everything in between. I am sure that some of the stories, or portions of many stories, will be similar to yours or that of your loved one, and hopefully they will offer you a clearer path to recovery.
- People **do** recover from bulimia and other disordered eating habits they may have. If you or a loved one is suffering with bulimia, the sooner the condition is recognized and acknowledged, the better the chances are of recovering and moving forward to live a full and satisfying life. To make that happen, you need to push past the myths, mystery, fear, and denial that surround bulimia and other eating disorders and realize that they are just that: **diseases**. They and the behaviors that characterize them are **not** you or your sister or your daughter or your son or your best friend. The bingeing and purging are separate from the person; they can be stopped, and the healing person can break through.

One reason why bulimia remains enveloped in secrecy, misconceptions, and feelings of shame and guilt is that both the disease and the motivation and mindset of the individuals who live with the disease are not well understood, not only by the family and friends of bulimics, but by bulimics themselves and indeed by many medical professionals as well. Adding to the confusion and mystery is the fact that bulimia is a multifaceted disease, which means there is no single cause, no single motivation, and no single treatment that can explain it away. Which means we have to dig a little deeper.

Myths about Bulimia

Let's start with some of the myths that surround bulimia. Belief in these ideas can be very damaging, as they can prevent bulimics from seeking help and discourage their loved ones from trying to help them.

- **It's all about food.** Wrong. Bingeing, purging, and starving are eating behaviors that individuals use in an attempt to solve or cope with their emotional problems. Although it is true that establishing healthy eating habits is a critical part of treatment of eating disorders, these efforts **will not be effective** unless the emotional issues are addressed and resolved. That is why a holistic approach that focuses on psychiatric help and incorporates other therapies is paramount, which I will talk about in chapter 6 on "Treatment."
- **Once you are bulimic, you will always be bulimic.** This is not true, reports Abigail H. Natenshon, PhD, an eating disorder specialist for more than thirty years and author of *When Your Child Has an Eating Disorder.* Research shows that when bulimia is detected early and treated effectively, 80 percent of patients recover. This percentage worsens, however, the longer one waits to seek professional help.
- **It's the parents' fault** when their children develop bulimia or other eating disorders. "Mea culpa" might be the most common phrase uttered by the parents of children who have bulimia or other eating disorders, but experts agree that this once-held belief is not so. I talk more about the causes of bulimia later in this chapter.

- **Bulimia only affects young girls.** Although the majority of people who have bulimia are young females, it is also true that an increasing number of women in their thirties, forties, and fifties are seeking help for bingeing, purging, and other disordered eating activities that they have been engaged in for decades. Another fact that dispels the myth is that bulimia and other eating disorder behavior is believed to occur in up to 15 percent of males. One group that is especially prone to abnormal eating behaviors is young males who are involved in sports that emphasize leanness and/or weight control, such as cross-country, wrestling, and gymnastics.
- **Most doctors are knowledgeable about eating disorders** and can accurately identify and effectively treat them. Unfortunately, this is far from the truth. This is why it is critically important to find a qualified professional to help you or your loved one. We discuss this issue in chapter 5.

"HUNGER OF AN OX"

To the outside world, Mavis looks like a normal, well-adjusted, responsible young woman. She graduated from the University of Chicago with a degree in business administration and works as an assistant manager at a nationally known bank. She's always well dressed, is at her desk before nine each morning, and gets "excellent" ratings on all her job reviews. To her colleagues and acquaintances, she appears self-confident and outgoing, and always has a ready smile for everyone, from the grocery clerk to the president of the bank. Away from the office she has a few friends, but she doesn't see them much because she says she's always "busy" with errands or taking a course in something like Italian or photography. Occasionally she goes out on a date, usually with someone a friend sets up, but there's "no one special," and at twenty-six she says she's happy to play the field for a while and is "too busy" to worry about romance.

But what keeps Mavis busy isn't Italian or photography or errands; it's bulimia. Since age 16, Mavis has been bingeing and purging, at least once a day in the beginning, and then progressively more often, sometimes inducing vomiting six or eight times a day. Mavis doesn't begin her day with a doughnut and coffee; she eats about two dozen doughnuts, or several bags of chocolate chip cookies or whatever other sweets she has stashed away and then washes it down with a 44-ounce diet soft drink from the corner convenience store on the way to work. Then she vomits it all up. Since her apartment is less than a half-mile away from her office, she goes home for lunch, binges and purges again, and returns to work.

The term "bulimia nervosa" literally means 'the hunger of an ox,' but the hunger Mavis and other bulimics experience is not one that can be satisfied by food. During a binge, Mavis says it's "like being in another world, a crazy, frantic world. I'm out of control, and it's terrifying." Once the binge is over, Mavis is driven by feelings of intense self-hatred to rid herself of the food by vomiting—the purging method practiced by the vast majority of bulimics. When the latest cycle of bingeing and purging is over, Mavis is filled with shame and disgust. She often swears she will not do it again, but she does, and the cycle goes on and on. The hunger she feels represents an emotional need that food cannot fulfill, but she says, she will still binge again. The smiles and self-assured face she wears for the world hide how Mavis really feels: scared, insecure, hopeless, and depressed.

So far, Mavis has kept her bulimia hidden from her family, friends, and coworkers. But she is paying an increasingly hard price for her secret. "Sometimes I spend most of a weekend bingeing and purging and sleeping it off," she says. "I have no social life, and I rarely see my friends. My family thinks I'm out with my friends every weekend, my friends think I'm with my family, and the truth is that I'm with food. I don't know how much longer I can hide what I'm doing, especially since my teeth are starting to look really bad, and I'm terrified to go to a dentist."

WHO DEVELOPS BULIMIA?

At one time, bulimia was first being seen in children 12 to 14 years old. As if developing this life-threatening disease at such an early age wasn't frightening enough, that average age of onset has now dropped to 9 to 12 years. The vast majority—85 to 90 percent—of those with bulimia are female, with some experts saying its prevalence among males is as low as 5 percent. Among males, those more likely to be bulimic are boys and men who are involved in sports that require or prefer them to "meet weight," such as wrestling, boxing, track and field, swimming, diving, and gymnastics. Among females, the pressure to be thin prevails in these same sports, as well as dance.

Another statistic that is especially interesting is that the number of women thirty or older who are bulimic appears to be increasing, although reliable data are not yet available. But if we look at some related data that reveal an obsession with weight and body image, those increasing numbers are no surprise. Research shows, for example, that 56 percent of women in midlife are dissatisfied with their body image and that more than 20% of women 70 and older are on a diet. At any one time, approximately 43 million women in the US are trying to lose weight and another 26 million are on a diet to help maintain their weight. Studies also show that 50 percent of women say eating causes them to feel guilty, and more than 90 percent are worried about their weight.

Although it is difficult to state with great certainty the numbers of people who suffer with eating disorders, it is especially challenging when it comes to bulimia because it is a disease that individuals practice in secret, and physical signs of the disease are often not apparent or are overlooked. People with bulimia also typically wait many years before they seek treatment—if indeed they do at all—or they may have the disease for many years before someone suspects there is a problem and confronts them with it. The average time a victim waits before getting treatment is 7 years! They try dieting first before discovering—if they ever do—that eating disorders are not about food.

The important point is that if you are bulimic or if you suspect a loved one has the disease, **now** is the time to act. The longer someone engages in bingeing and purging, the more engrained the behaviors become and the more emotional and physical damage accumulates, including damage to the teeth and mouth.

CAUSES AND TRIGGERS OF BULIMIA

Twiggy is back (if you're too young to know who she was, picture Calista Flockhart or Nicole Ritchie with a British accent), and she's brought with her an entourage of other waif-like creatures from movies, television, sports, and fashion. The pressure to be thin and to sport designer-labeled clothing on hanger-like shoulders is pervasive and dangerous. There is even more pressure for these young girls to grow up faster than any other generation in history. Girls as young as five and six years old are picking out their own designer clothes and dictating to their parents what they will wear. These five-year-olds-going-on-thirty children, as well as prepubescent and young teens, hear about and see pictures of young TV and movie idols and fashion models who are dangerously thin and then try to imitate the look. One young mother whose seven-year-old daughter, Madison, was purging after her meals says she overheard Madison say to a friend, "Don't wear *those* pants, they make you look fat. I'll never be fat. I won't, I just won't."

Although few can deny that the media has a role in encouraging women to be thin, it is far too simplistic to claim they are the only or even the primary cause of eating disorder behaviors. Experts generally agree that bulimia and other eating disorders are caused by a combination of environmental, social, and biological factors. Current research is uncovering some interesting findings in these areas, which will hopefully help us find effective ways to prevent these disorders. For now, however, let's look at the factors beyond social pressures to be thin that experts believe contribute to the development of bulimia and how they may be a part of your life or that of a loved one.

Blaming Biology

Research into genetic factors in bulimia is in its infancy, but some intriguing results are turning up. Recent studies suggest, for example, that genetics play a significant role in predisposing some people to traits such as perfectionism, anxiety, and obsessive-compulsive behaviors and thoughts, which are typical characteristics of people who have bulimia and other eating disorders. Thus if you inherit a tendency for these characteristics, you may be a higher risk of developing these disorders.

Family history also has a role. If your mother or sister had bulimia, you are four times more likely to also develop the disease, and when it comes to anorexia, the likelihood you will also have the disease jumps to twelve times if your mother or sister also suffered with it. Since approximately half of all people who suffer with bulimia also engage in anorexic behaviors at least occasionally, these are important factors to remember.

Other researchers have evidence that levels of autoantibodies against a specific hormone (alpha-melanocycle-stimulating hormone) have a role in bulimia and anorexia, as they influence appetite and stress response. Such information is important because it may eventually lead experts to find better ways to treat and even prevent eating disorders.

A chemical in the brain known as serotonin may also play a role in bulimia. Serotonin is a neurotransmitter (a substance that facilitates the transmission of nerve signals), which is involved in satiety. Some bulimics have low serotonin levels, and given the hormone's possible role in satiety, such levels may contribute to the persistence of bingeing: because they don't feel full, they continue to binge.

Certain other substances in the brain also may be involved. A study found that brain hormones called cytokines were threefold higher in bulimics than in controls, while other research showed that the hormone vasopressin was higher in the fluid surrounding the brain of bingeing patients with bulimia or anorexia and in patients with major depression, but not in healthy controls.

It's important to know that bingeing and purging can change brain chemistry and thus perpetuate the desire to continue these behaviors. Think, for example, about what we commonly refer to as "comfort foods," such as ice cream, macaroni and cheese, French fries, and doughnuts. These high fat, simple carbohydrate foods temporarily activate brain chemicals (e.g., serotonin) that suppress feelings of anxiety and depression and produce feelings of calm and euphoria. Bingeing, purging, and starving can produce these same feelings, which suggests that people with bulimia and other eating disorders use food to help them cope with depression, painful memories and emotions, and everyday stress.

Even more reason to nip bulimia in the bud as early as possible is evidence that bingeing, purging, and starving can have lasting, detrimental effects on the brain. We know from magnetic resonance imaging (MRI) studies that the brain continues to develop until we reach our early twenties; especially the regions that are responsible for helping us manage emotions, predict consequences, and plan ahead. (Note: This is a major reason why teenagers have difficulties in these three areas; the regions of the brain responsible for these functions have not yet fully matured. If you're a parent, this may or may not make you feel better, but at least it may partly explain your child's behavior.) Eating disorder behaviors can thus have a devastating impact on how these brain regions develop. Unfortunately, if you continue these behaviors beyond the early twenties, they also continue to cause harm to brain chemistry and functioning.

Trauma

In 2005, a Harvard University case-control study (one in which people with the condition under study are compared with people who are free of the condition) provided evidence to support what many experts believe to be true: that trauma experienced early in life (childhood and/or adolescence) is a risk factor for eating disorders. The Harvard study looked at women 36 to 44 years of age who had been diagnosed with bulimia, anorexia, or binge-eating disorder and found that those who reported childhood physical abuse were twice as likely to have an eating disorder than those who had not been abused. Similarly, women who had been both physically and sexually abused had a nearly fourfold increased risk of meeting the DSM-IV criteria for an eating disorder. Although the study did not study women who had purging disorder as a diagnosis, it seems safe to assume that the findings would apply to this eating disorder as well.

Learned Behavior

Children (and adults) learn through imitation, and typically their role models are their parents. Although it would be most helpful if children were born with a gene that was programmed for optimal eating habits, lack of such a gene makes it necessary for parents to serve as role models when it comes to healthy eating behaviors and attitudes about body image and weight. When parents themselves have an eating disorder or have difficulties with these issues, they can unwittingly pass along distorted ideas about food, weight, and body image to their children. Research shows, for example, that children who have an anorexic mother display higher rates of depression, whining, and distorted eating habits. Women with bulimia have reported that as children, they can remember times when one or both parents would make innocent comments or engage in behaviors that they now recognize as being instrumental in their attitudes about weight and food.

"My mother would often say, 'I'd rather die than be bigger than a size six,' and then fast several days a week to make sure she stayed a six," explains Suzanne, a thirty-one-year-old recovering bulimic. "I remember sitting at the dinner table, choking down my food while my mother sat there with a glass of water. My father never said a word, and I always felt like such a pig for eating while my mother just sat there, nursing her water."

This is not to say that Suzanne's parents or anyone's parents are responsible for causing their son or daughter to develop an eating disorder, but it does say that a parent's attitudes, behaviors, and beliefs have an impact on a child and may play a role in triggering an eating disorder in a child who is susceptible because of other contributing factors, including environmental, biological, and genetic.

Life Changes

For some people, significant losses or transitions in their lives that cause emotional turmoil they are unable to deal with adequately can trigger bulimia. Puberty, going away to college, divorce, death of a loved one, moving away from treasured friends, starting a new job-all of these situations have something in common: varying degrees of uncertainty, anxiety, risk, and/or loss of control, and the ability to trigger distorted eating. Indeed, to deal with situations over which they have little or no control, some people reach out for something they believe they can control—eating. The irony is, for some people the tables are turned and eating controls them.

Dieting

It may sound overly simplistic, but the act of dieting itself can be a trigger for bingeing and purging. Consider this: when people diet, they often are chronically hungry. This can cause them to overeat, feel guilty, and then purge to get rid of the calories. This is how Glenda first started to binge and purge. "It seemed obvious to me," says the now-recovered thirty-four-year-old insurance adjuster. "I had tried so many diets, and none of them worked. I needed to lose about 25 pounds, but I kept losing and regaining the same ten pounds for years. One day I weighed myself after getting through a very hard week when I was very careful about everything I ate. I was sure I had lost some weight, but the scale said I had actually gained a pound. I was so upset, I sat down and ate an entire bag of Famous Amos chocolate chip cookies." Horrified by what she had done, she remembered reading about a woman who said she vomited after overeating as a way to keep her weight down. "So I tried it, and even though I hated the thought of vomiting, I was relieved to get rid of the calories. After that, I just became numb and it became easier."

One problem with dieting is that some people allow themselves to get so hungry; it's nearly impossible for them not to binge. The healthiest way to eat, whether you are trying to lose weight or just maintain your weight, is to eat appropriate amounts of nutritious food when you feel hungry and not to overeat.

Psychological Triggers

Because bulimia is a disease about emotions, psychological factors are always a part of the picture, and therefore it is necessary to identify and then either treat them (in cases of depression, anxiety disorder, or obsessive-compulsive disorder, for example) or learn to modify them (having unrealistic expectations of oneself; perfectionistic).

Some bulimics binge and purge as ways to deal with anger. Because they are unable to express their anger in a healthy or constructive way, and because they are afraid of disapproval or criticism, they direct their anger inward, stuffing themselves and then purging.

Never underestimate the power of a sad movie, according to a research team at Harvard. They found that bingeing increases among bulimics when they watch sad movies or movies that threaten their self-esteem. The investigators theorize that bulimics have much less resilience to such stimulators than normal controls and that they act out their subconscious aggressions with bingeing and purging.

Fear is a great motivator, and for bulimics it can be very damaging. Bulimics want and need to be in control of themselves and their lives all the time, but in the real world this isn't possible, so they take control of their food. To the outside world they may appear strong and confident, but inside they are afraid and feel powerless, weak, and resentful. When you combine this need for control with the tendency to be perfectionistic, you have a very powerful, unrealistic, and ultimately damaging combination that helps perpetuate the cycle of bingeing and purging.

Sports or Work Pressures

Researchers have found what many people have suspected for some time: People who are involved in certain sports and careers, such as gymnastics, track and field, wrestling, dance (especially ballet), modeling, and acting, are at higher risk of eating disorders such as bulimia, because weight and appearance are intimately associated with success in these endeavors. In one large Norwegian study, for example, more than 1,600 male and female elite athletes were compared with controls and evaluated for the presence of eating disorders. Eating disorders were identified in 13.5 percent of the athletes and only 4.6 percent of controls, and they were more common among females than males.

When the individuals involved are children and adolescents, the pressure from coaches, parents, and peers to be thin or to lose weight can be especially powerful and damaging. Responsible adults need to ensure that young people are not being allowed to endanger their future and their lives by encouraging or supporting disordered eating behaviors.

Pro-Bulimia and Pro-Anorexic Websites

At any one time, there are hundreds of pro-bulimia (known as "pro-mia") and pro-anorexic ("pro-ana") web sites on the internet. Although these sites are not a cause of bulimia or other eating disorders, they can trigger distorted eating behaviors and perhaps even more alarming, they support, encourage, and validate bingeing, purging, and starving. People who visit these websites—mostly young, impressionable young women—are lulled by the sense of community and acceptance they offer.

The message these websites give is potentially lethal; that is, that bulimia and anorexia are *not* illnesses but instead a way of life, a life choice that people have a right to make if they want to. These sites make eating disorders seem chic and glamorous, and they often display pictures of bulimic and anorexic celebrities, such as Nicole Ritchie and Kate Moss, as examples of "success." They also offer suggestions on how to deceive family and friends, plus offer harmful tips and techniques on how to lose weight. Even though many search engines have banned these websites, they continue to exist and thrive. Efforts by concerned individuals and organizations such as the National Association of Anorexia Nervosa and Associated Disorders to shut down or ban these sites continues.

BULIMIA: SIGNS AND SYMPTOMS

One of the most common questions concerned individuals ask about bulimia is: Are there any early warning signs? The answer is yes, but they often are not obvious. Many parents and friends of bulimics comment that they didn't know their child or friend had an eating disorder because they didn't know what to look for. "She didn't look too thin" people will often say. But did you know, for example, that most people with bulimia are close to normal weight, and that 15 percent are obese? Therefore, unlike anorexia nervosa, bulimia is largely a "hidden" disease when it comes to signs associated with body weight. That's one reason why we need to look for other clues, in personality, behavior, and physical signs, all of which I discuss here.

Personality Traits of People with Bulimia

"Looking back, I can see now that Rachael showed many of the traits of a person who could develop bulimia," says her mother, Susan. She sits alone in her Oregon living room, looking at childhood pictures of her daughter, who took her own life at age nineteen after a four-year battle with bulimia and anorexia. "If I had known what those traits are, and then pieced them together with some of her behaviors, I may have more easily recognized that something was wrong. But who knew? She never lost a lot of weight. She had so many wonderful characteristics; she was such a caring, loving person. We didn't realize how tormented she was deep inside."

The degree of turmoil Susan refers to is certainly not the same for every person who suffers with bulimia, but there are some characteristics and behaviors that are common among people who develop the disease. Not all of them are easy to identify, nor are they all considered to be "negative" traits. One hallmark underlying characteristic, however, is this: very low self-esteem based to an excessive degree on the individual's perception of her/his body weight and shape. Susan remembers how Rachael was constantly critical about her weight, always saying she was "too fat," even though she was actually thin for her height, and often weighing herself ten times a day.

Hindsight, as they say, is 20/20, so a little foresight is in order. Here I've provided two lists: one consists of behavioral and emotional signs and symptoms of bulimia, another of physical ones. We will discuss the items in these lists again in chapter 4, but for now you should familiarize yourself with their contents so you can begin to better understand bulimia and help yourself or a loved one on the road to recovery.

Emotional and Behavioral Signs and Symptoms

Generally, people who develop bulimia exhibit some or many of the following emotional and behavioral signs and symptoms.

- Highly sensitive at an early age.
- Feels responsible for traumas or hardships in the family, such as divorce, a sick or disabled sibling, or death of a family member.
- Harbors a sense of doom about life in general and/or about specific aspects of life
- Altruistic, selfless
- Has great difficulty expressing his or her emotions. It is common for people with bulimia to be truly baffled when asked how they feel about something. Peggy's comments are typical. "My therapists would give me a situation and then ask me, 'How does that make you feel?' And my mind would go blank. I wouldn't know what to say. I would get an overwhelming urge to binge at that moment, and I wanted to scream at them, 'Don't ask me that question.' I couldn't identify or even name my feelings, because I didn't know how to access them. I was waiting for someone to tell me what I was feeling. We're still

working on this in therapy, and I've gotten much better naming how I feel about things."

- Has great difficulty expressing his or her own needs or desires. People with bulimia typically believe they have no right to have desires and needs. Their self-esteem is so low; they often don't value themselves enough to allow themselves to feel pleasure or joy.
- Obsesses about weight, food, and body image. A person with bulimia may weigh herself a dozen or more times a day, read food labels obsessively, or keep a diary of every calorie and fat gram she consumes.
- Has difficulty making decisions and will defer to others' needs or desires. When asked what she wants to do (e.g., go to a movie or stay at home), she'll say, "I don't care, what do you want to do?"
- Severe self-criticism. Bulimics may berate themselves for being "stupid," or "too fat," or "never good enough."
- Excessive desire for privacy, usually in the bathroom and/or bedroom
- Isolates or withdraws from family and friends
- Lie or steal to get food. Claudia, a twenty-one-year-old college student, says she used to go to four different food stores, buying the cheapest cookies, doughnuts, and other sweets she could find, and then bring them all back to her dorm room. "By the second year of college, I couldn't afford to keep buying a lot of food, so I lied to my parents," she says. "I told them I needed money to fix my car. That worked once, but then about four months later I really needed to fix my car, and they said it wasn't worth fixing again, so they wouldn't send any money. So I lied again: I sold the car for a thousand dollars and used the money for food, but I told my parents that I got only two hundred for the car."
- Has strange food- or eating-related behaviors, such as cutting food into tiny pieces, arranging food in patterns or separating it on the plate
- Makes excessive food purchases. Bulimics spend a lot of money and time acquiring food. Depending on how much access they have to transportation, grocery stores, and money, some bulimics travel from store to store, spreading out their purchases so they don't look suspicious.

Physical Signs and Symptoms

Tori is a thirty-eight-year-old recovering bulimic who got some shocking news from her doctor a few days after she fell off her bike and broke her arm: she had osteoporosis, and in fact her bone density was like that of a seventy-year-old woman. Why? Her sixteen-plus years of bingeing and purging had left her severely deficient in calcium and other bone-promoting nutrients and thus placed her at high risk of fractures.

Osteoporosis is just one of the many "hidden" consequences of bulimia, hidden because this disease largely takes its toll internally. But not all of the physical consequences of bulimia are so well hidden. Tori, like many people with bulimia, also displayed telltale signs in her mouth. In Tori's case, those signs included swollen gums, eroded tooth enamel, and several rotting teeth. Tori had avoided going to a dentist for several years because she was extremely embarrassed about her teeth and afraid that her dentist would know she had been purging. Tori did eventually go to three different dentists to take care of her dental problems, and she lied to each one, telling one that she had gastric reflux disease, and the other two that she ate a lot of citrus and brushed excessively.

In addition to osteoporosis, some other physical effects of bulimia (many of which are hidden) are listed here. An in-depth discussion of many of the physical and medical consequences of bingeing and purging is in chapter 3.

- anemia
- cardiovascular problems, including irregular heart beat, weakened heart muscle, heart failure, low pulse, low blood pressure
- dehydration
- low electrolyte (potassium, magnesium, sodium) levels
- gastrointestinal difficulties, including constipation, irregular bowel movements, bloating, diarrhea, abdominal cramping, bloody vomit, stomach pain, ulcers
- irregular or absent menstrual cycle
- dental problems. We take a close look at the impact of bulimia on oral health in chapter 4.

- dizziness
- Abrasions or scars on the back of the hands or knuckles
- Dry skin, nails, and/or hair
- Torn or ruptured esophagus or stomach
- Candida infections

A DANGEROUS LIAISON: BULIMIA AND ANOREXIA

How often do individuals have both bulimia and anorexia together? It's a question that hadn't crossed my mind when I first became actively involved in helping people who have bulimia. In fact, I thought the two eating disorders were basically separate entities. In reality, however, it's estimated that 40 to 60 percent of bulimics also engage in some anorexic behavior, either occasionally or regularly. Knowing that this type of crossover or combination behavior may be a part of your life or that of your loved one is important if healing is to occur. Therefore, let's take a look at anorexia nervosa and its role and impact on people who have bulimia.

Diagnosis: Anorexia Nervosa

According to the *Diagnostic and Statistical Manual of Mental Disorders IV,* four factors are included in a clinical diagnosis of the disease. These are guidelines only, as not everyone with the condition experiences all of them.

- Refuses to maintain body weight at or above a figure that is minimally normal for the individual's age and height. Typically a person is referred to as anorexic if body weight is 15 percent or more below normal.
- Maintains an abnormal response to body weight or shape (e.g., individuals see or believe they are fat when they are not) and/or believes that weight or shape determines self-worth ("I'm never thin enough, I'm never good enough"), and/or denies the seriousness of current low body weight
- Has an intense, irrational fear of gaining weight or becoming fat. People with anorexia often even forego drinking water because they say it makes them heavy.

- Experiences a lack of at least three consecutive menstrual cycles (among females who have not yet gone through menopause). This happens because the body stops producing enough estrogen for menstruation to occur.

Experts have also identified two subtypes of anorexia. In the *restricting type,* which is the category most people are familiar with, individuals lose weight by severely reducing their food intake, fasting, or exercising excessively to work off calories. Many people with this type of anorexia engage in two or all three of these activities. In the *binge-eating/purging type,* individuals restrict their food intake but also binge and/or purge, either by vomiting or abusing diuretics, laxatives, or enemas.

Thus you can see that it is not unusual for individuals to crisscross the lines between various types of eating disorders and behaviors. A bulimic who also sometimes restricts food intake, for example, is similar to a binge-eating/purging type of anorexic, although bulimia is still the "main" disorder.

I present these definitions merely to make you aware of the different types of behaviors that can occur in people who have bulimia, and to impress upon you that bulimia and anorexia are not black and white issues. Bulimia, and indeed all eating disorders, are multifaceted conditions that require multidisciplinary treatment and management approaches that take into consideration each person's unique personality and circumstances. There are, however, some traits, beliefs, and behaviors that are common to anorexia, bulimia, and purging disorder, and understanding them can help you—either a person with bulimia or the loved one of a person with the disease—to overcome the challenges of the disease.

Characteristics of People with Anorexia

People who are anorexic typically are obsessed with food, and often make it a point to know the calorie and fat content of foods. Many of them confine themselves to a very limited list of foods they will even consider eating, and when they do eat them they frequently perform rituals around them. Ruth, for example, was a bulimic and an anorexic who occasionally did what her husband, Marty, called "weird food play." He explains:

"We had been married for about three months when I first noticed my wife's strange food behaviors. Ruth would cut her food into very tiny pieces, arrange them on her plate in some sort of elaborate pattern, and then systematically take one piece at a time and chew each piece very slowly. It would take her such a long time to eat, and I'd always be done way ahead of her. Then once I was done, she could throw away what was left on her plate, or feed it to the dogs. At the time I didn't have any idea that she was even bulimic, even though I found out later that she had been bingeing and purging for more than five years, so it started before we were married. No one in her family knew she had eating disorders."

Similar to bulimics, people with anorexia tend to be perfectionists who are also highly intelligent and driven to succeed. They view their ability to control their food intake as a sign of great self-control and an accomplishment. When they "fail" to maintain that control—if they are forced to eat or believe they have eaten too much—they are filled with self-loathing.

PURGING DISORDER

Study results reported in December 2005 suggest that an eating disorder called purging disorder (PD), in which individuals purge frequently but do not binge, is more common than bulimia and anorexia combined. If this is true, then millions more people than originally realized are living a life of secrecy and are at risk of serious health problems associated with purging. According to Dr. Pamela K. Keel, who headed the study at the University of Iowa, the questionnaires used to screen for bulimia probably miss people who have PD because they don't binge and they are usually of normal weight.

They are people like Rita, a twenty-four-year-old mother of one who also works part-time as a receptionist at a real estate office. "I've been purging for about five years," she says, "but I never binge. Throwing up is the only way I can keep my weight down. If I didn't purge at least once a day, I'd be huge. I just can't control my weight any other way."

Unfortunately, this kind of thinking is not uncommon among people with purging disorder or bulimia. That's not to say that purging disorder and bulimia are exactly alike. In her study Dr. Keel found that when she compared women who had PD with those who had bulimia, those with PD were less impulsive about eating and less impulsive overall, and also reported less hunger. Both groups of women, however, had similar degrees of body image disturbance.

Although there is still a lot we don't know about purging disorder, the fact that it exists and likely affects millions of people is all the reason we need to pay close attention to possible signs and symptoms among friends and loved ones and to offer them help while we wait for more research to be done. We look at purging disorder again in chapters 3 and 4.

BOTTOM LINE

It is often said that we should not confuse the message with the messenger, nor should we confuse an individual with his or her behavior. Indeed, we are first and foremost physical, emotional, spiritual beings, not "the things we do." Bulimia can be a scary thing, both for the people who are in its throes and for those who care about them. But it is a "thing" that can be shed, not like a coat, but more like a layer of skin that some people "grow" to help them cope with painful emotional issues. Underneath this skin is a caring person who deserves to be free of this burden.

That burden is both physical and emotional, and it is the topic we discuss in the next chapter. A deeper understanding of the physical and emotional factors that make up bulimia will help you in your efforts to shed this disease for yourself or others.

CHAPTER 3

BODY AND SOUL:
THE PHYSICAL AND PSYCHOLOGICAL
IMPACT OF BULIMIA

"What are you thinking? What do you feel?" Most people would consider these to be routine, benign questions, yet for people who suffer with bulimia, they can invoke unexpected, highly unsatisfying, yet very revealing responses. "I don't know." "My thoughts scare me." "I try not to think." "I'm not sure what I feel." "I don't feel anything."

At first you may think, how can people not know what they feel? Is something wrong with them? Is it true they don't feel anything?

The answers are yes, no, and no, but I want to focus on the last response. We know this is not true, and in fact, quite the opposite is the case. People with bulimia feel a great deal. They are often overwhelmed with emotional pain, with thoughts that frighten, anger, and confuse them. They can become anxious, even experience panic attacks, when these feelings overcome them. And they have found a way, albeit a self-destructive and distorted way, to cope with these negative emotions and feelings, and that way is bingeing and purging. These activities then take a physical toll on their body, resulting in many short- and long-term consequences and sometimes even threatening their lives.

One of the biggest barriers that prevent family, friends, medical professionals, and other concerned individuals from reaching out and helping those who suffer with bulimia and other eating disorders is fear, and that fear originates in a lack of understanding what goes on in the mind of bulimics.

People with bulimia are in pain. They want to rid themselves of the pain, but they don't know how to do it in a healthy way. The ways they have chosen cause them shame and guilt, so they become secretive and try to hide their behaviors. All of this makes it a challenge to connect with bulimics and help them rid themselves of destructive habits and replace them with healthy ones. A challenge—but it can be done.

In this chapter I explore the complicated world of the bulimic mind and the impact the thoughts and emotions of bulimics have on their emotional/spiritual and physical well-being. I am grateful to those men and women who have been willing to open up their hearts and share their feelings about bulimia and what goes on in their mind. Expressing these emotions can be very painful, even though doing so is an essential part of the healing and recovery process.

THE POWER OF MIND

If there is one "enemy" of the bulimic, it is not food; it's the mind.

"My mind just takes over," says Paul, a twenty-one-year-old part-time college student and part-time software developer. "Every time I go on a binge and then purge, I tell myself that I won't binge and purge again, that I have control of the situation. A day may go by, even two, but then the mind takes over. It sneaks in and before I know it, I'm bingeing again. I'm out of control, and I don't even know how it happens."

What goes on in the mind of a bulimic? "You don't want to know," says Misty, who admitted that she had contemplated committing suicide several times. She had just been released from a residential treatment facility and was living at home with her parents temporarily. She planned to return to her junior year of college after taking a semester off to "learn how to think and feel again."

"I wasn't doing well in school because I couldn't concentrate," she says. "I had always been a good student in high school, but once the bulimia took over when I was a freshman in college, my grades started to slip. The more trouble I had concentrating and studying, the more I worried and had panic attacks and the more I binged and purged. It was a vicious cycle. I felt like an emotional time bomb, ready to explode any second. Binging and purging defused it, but only temporarily. I wanted to die."

In a fortunate, but also unfortunate turn of events, Misty was arrested one night early in her junior year for shoplifting twenty bags of candy from a grocery store. "I was scared out of my mind," she says, and terribly embarrassed that she had to call her parents to bail her out of jail. The whole experience shocked her into admitting she had an eating problem—which her parents had not realized up to that point—and that she needed help.

Bulimics experience a broad spectrum of emotions that can range in severity from mild to severe and back again. These feelings are the driving force behind the disease and the physical toll they take throughout the body. That is why healing the emotional turmoil and psychological pain is the number one goal of treatment of bulimia and purging disorder. **Unless the emotional pain is identified and managed in a satisfactory way, bulimic behavior will not be resolved.** Let's look at some of the feelings and emotional challenges bulimics live with every day. One thing I believe you'll notice is that there is considerable overlap of emotions, until sometimes it is impossible to separate them from each other. Control, for example, is intimately related to the need to be perfect, but it is also tied to a sense of guilt and self-disgust when the bulimic believes he or she has failed to be perfect or maintain control. Thus the emotional landscape of bulimia is a complex one indeed.

Need to Control

It's paradoxical that the bulimic's intense desire to be in control and the control he or she attempts to have over food ultimately results in a complete loss of control—bingeing and purging. The need for control doesn't stop with food or with how their body looks, however. Bulimics also want to control their family, friends, and work environment—basically everything around them. They feel responsible for everyone else's happiness, but they neglect their own. They want to make the world a better place, and when they can't, they berate themselves with self-hate and negative thoughts (see "Self-Hate" and "Negative Voices" below).

"Feeling like I was out of control was one of the worst feelings," says Roberta, who has been in recovery for more than three years.

"I needed to control everything around me, and when I couldn't, I went crazy. I binged. It got very scary, because I was beginning to be overcome by the urge to binge while I was at work, and I couldn't do it there. That's when I realized I needed help, but I still had this illusion that I could control my actions. Naturally, I couldn't, and it took me almost a year before I went to a therapist and found a treatment program that worked."

The overwhelming feeling that one needs to be in control is a hallmark of bulimia and anorexia. Bulimics are typically strong-willed, capable individuals, but inside they often feel weak, defeated, ineffective, and victimized. Similar to an anorexic, a bulimic tries to control her food intake, but the difference is that the bulimic is overcome by a desire to eat and gives in to it by going on a binge. In the mind of the bulimic, she is a failure because she has lost control, and so she purges. The cycle is then repeated again and again until she gets help.

Need to be Perfect

Along with the need to control everything in their lives, bulimics also tend to be perfectionists. Perfectionists are overly critical of their performance and have an excessive need for approval. According to a study conducted by the Virginia Institute for Psychiatric and Behavioral Genetics at Virginia Commonwealth University and published in *American Journal of Psychiatry,* perfectionists are driven by fear, whereas high achievers are driven by a desire to achieve. The study also found that negative reactions to making mistakes and a tendency to believe ones mistakes are personal failures are perfectionist characteristics that are most associated with bulimia and anorexia among women.

Very often, bulimics are on the honor roll in school, excel at a sport or hobby, and are always striving to "do better." They may be able to forgive others for not being perfect, but they can't forgive themselves. Similarly, they may find it easy to congratulate a friend or relative for an achievement, but if they were to achieve the same thing, they would view it in a negative way.

Perhaps the most significant finding of the study is that there appears to be something unique about perfectionism that increases the risk for bulimia and anorexia, but for now exactly what that "something" is, is not clear. What researchers believe they do know, however, is that young girls who show evidence of being highly perfectionistic and who berate or punish themselves for what they perceive to be personal failures can and should be helped to be less hard on themselves and to set more realistic goals and expectations for themselves. A significant part of the psychotherapy for bulimics involves changing their negative ways of thinking and adopting positive, self-supporting thoughts.

Out of Body Experience

"Sometimes I think I'm going crazy," says Joycelyn, a twenty-five-year-old assistant manager, who has been bingeing and purging for nearly six years. She says she sometimes has an "out of body" experience when she binges. This is not uncommon, especially during the early stages of bulimia, when individuals may feel extremely anxious or frantic, completely out of control, when they binge.

"It's like someone else is stuffing all that food inside herself," says Joycelyn. "I don't feel anything, I don't want to feel anything. At the same time, it's scary because I think I'm cracking up." Once the binge is done, the bulimic usually experiences depression and feelings of self-hatred and disgust. These feelings make it difficult for bulimics to admit they need help and so they are very reluctant to seek it or accept it from others.

Low Self-esteem

Hand-in-hand with control and perfectionism is low self-esteem. Self-esteem is inherent not only in bulimia but also in all eating disorders, and so it's important to have a clear understanding of what it is. According to Peter H. Silverstone at the University of Alberta, Canada, self-esteem is "the sense of contentment and self-acceptance that stems from a person's appraisal of their own worth, significance, attractiveness, competence and ability to satisfy their aspirations."

Given that definition, it's not hard to spot low self-esteem in many bulimics. Kirsten, a thirty-year-old claims adjuster is an example:

"I feel like I'm the lowest of the low, a worthless human being," says Kirsten during one of her group therapy sessions. Kirsten had admitted to her husband that she was bulimic, and for the past two months she has been seeing a therapist for group and one-on-one sessions twice a week. "It's really difficult to get over this feeling, hard to climb out of this hole I'm in," she says. "My husband tells me that I'm great, that he loves me, that I'm the best thing in his life, but I'm having a real hard time believing it. But I want to get better. Sometimes I think I can; other times I'm not so sure. I'm just taking it one day at a time."

Bulimics believe that when they "fail" at being perfect, they need to punish themselves or that they don't' deserve to be happy or to have good things. They have no confidence in their abilities, that they are significant to others, or that they can achieve goals. Their perception of themselves, physically and emotionally, is distorted. A bulimic may look at a thin person and say, "I wish I was as skinny as he is" or "I could never be as smart as she is" when in reality he is thinner and she is just as smart. The reason bulimics have such a difficult time seeing their own good qualities, especially when they compare themselves to others, is that they have very low self-esteem.

Self-Hate

One of the many emotions that plagues people with bulimia is self-hate, which is related to guilt, shame, and depression. "The amount of self-hatred is incredible," says twenty-nine-year-old Stacey, who battled bulimia and anorexia for more than ten years before she sought help in a residential facility. "I so wanted to die and I often thought about suicide, but I didn't want to upset my parents and sister by killing myself. Sometimes I think that's the only thing that prevented me from doing it. But every day I would look in the mirror and tell myself how disgusting I was. I really hated myself and what I was doing. Yet I didn't feel like I could stop."

Bulimics are disgusted with their distorted eating habits and purging, and they also self-hate because they believe they are weak, too fat, worthless, and not deserving of happiness. Stacey struggled with all of these feelings while trying to hide her bulimia from her family and friends.

"My mother was always inviting me over for dinner," says Stacey, "and I hated to go because purging was difficult there. Otherwise, I was able to hide the bulimia for many years, but once I started purging three or more times a day, I was often weak and very fatigued. I told my mother and sister that I had chronic fatigue syndrome, and they seemed to believe me, at least for a while. I hated myself for lying to them, but I felt I had to. Eventually my teeth got so bad I couldn't hide them any longer. Even though I was ashamed to go to a dentist, I got an abscess and had to make an appointment. He didn't confront me the first time I went, but on my second visit he talked to me about bulimia. He showed me the telltale signs of bulimia in my mouth and said my teeth would only get much worse, that I would lose many of them, if I continued bingeing and purging. That really scared me, and I finally agreed to get help."

Today, after more than a year since she left residential treatment, Stacey is pursuing a career in elementary education, has taken up rock climbing, and attends support group meetings several times a month to help keep her on track. The first thing she did after leaving treatment was start restoration work on her smile, and she's happy to report that it's "sparkling."

Guilt

Feelings of guilt can overcome bulimics for several reasons. One is the guilt they feel when they believe they haven't met the expectations of others or they've failed to meet their own expectations. Carl, a seventeen-year-old high school student who was on the school gymnastics team, had begun purging to keep his weight down. But this once-star athlete began to perform poorly as he got deeper and deeper into bulimia.

"I felt I was letting the team down," he said. "The worse I felt, the more I binged and purged. I let down the team in a statewide competition, and I felt so guilty I couldn't even go to school for a few days. And I was spending that time bingeing and purging at home while my parents were at work." Fortunately, Carl's coach suspected something was wrong and confronted the athlete with his suspicions. Carl was able to get help, and today he competes with his college team, free of bulimia.

Depression and Anxiety

It is estimated that up to 63 percent of people with bulimia also suffer with major depression. Some eating disorder specialists believe every bulimic suffers with depression. Certainly, many bulimics report having to battle with mood swings, feelings of hopelessness, lack of interest in activities and people that used to interest them, and sleep problems, all of which are characteristics of depression. Research also suggests that anxiety is fairly common (36% in one study), as are personality disorders, substance abuse (alcohol, prescription drugs, illegal drugs), and obsessive-compulsive disorder.

Results of a recent study can help mental health professionals as they treat bulimia. The study evaluated nearly 1,000 teenagers with bulimia and found that a lower level form of depression, known as dysthymia, is common among bulimics and may even predispose them to the eating disorder. Unlike major depression, which can resolve even if untreated, dysthymia is a chronic form of depression that often lasts for decades, with the average length of an episode being more than ten years. Researcher Marisol Perez, of Texas A&M University, reports that the chronic nature of dysthymia, compared with major depression, makes it more likely to be associated with bulimia, which is characterized by chronic low self-esteem. Therefore, psychiatric treatment should focus on this chronic form of depression rather than major depression in some patients.

Secrecy, Deception, and Stealing

Another hallmark of bulimia is secrecy. Because bulimics feel appalled and guilty about their binging and purging behaviors, they are highly secretive about their disease. In order to maintain their secret, they sometimes lie and deceive family, friends, and coworkers. When asked whether they have eaten lunch, for example, they may lie to avoid having to eat, or they may sneak or hide food in their room so they can binge on it later. They also hide their excessive use of laxatives, diuretics, and diet pills.

Some bulimics are like Misty (whom you read about earlier in this chapter) who become so overwhelmed by anxiety and panic that they steal food, laxatives, or diet pills to "support" their habit. Research shows that 65 to 67 percent of people with an eating disorder engage in kleptomania. It is important to understand that although bulimics are secretive, and they may lie, cheat, and even steal, **they don't do these things because they are bad people.** In fact, the deception, lying, or stealing bulimics engage in may help them maintain a feeling of control, but they also usually feel very guilty and a strong sense of self-disgust about doing it, which further feeds into the vicious cycle of bingeing and purging.

Negative Voices

Steve admits that when his daughter first mentioned the "negative voices" in her head, he was frightened. "I was afraid she had schizophrenia," he says. "I didn't understand, and at the same time I wanted so much to help her but didn't know how." Many bulimics talk about the negative self-talk and thoughts that go racing through their head, which some refer to as negative voices. It's important to remember that these voices come from within; they are self-talk, not voices from other people or entities. So although Steve's concern is understandable, his fears about schizophrenia are unfounded. (Note: Occasionally, bulimics hear actual voices, similar to what a schizophrenic hears, but in this case they are usually caused by dehydration or extreme malnutrition. A physician should address such auditory hallucinations immediately.)

Tabitha, a hair stylist who has been in recovery for two years after suffering with bulimia for nearly ten of her twenty-eight years, explains. "Just imagine all your thoughts about yourself are negative," she says, "and they just keep going through your mind. You're constantly putting yourself down, always telling yourself that you're no good, that you don't deserve to feel good, and the only way to get rid of all the negative voices is to focus your attention on food and weight, on eating and purging."

One of the goals of psychotherapy is to help bulimics conquer the voices and learn to love themselves for the caring individuals that they are. As destructive and negative as the voices are, some bulimics say that stopping them can be frightening too. "In some strange way, the voices are a friend," says Tabitha. "Having bulimia is an isolating thing, and the voices are sometimes our only friend, even though they aren't good friends."

If you are the friend or loved one of a bulimic, the best thing you can do is offer the bulimic love, positive reinforcement, and encouragement. For some ideas on how to handle negative voices, see chapter 5, where I talk about the types of things you should and should not say to someone who is suffering with bulimia.

PHYSICAL IMPACT

The physical consequences of bingeing and purging are real, serious, and potentially deadly, as has been demonstrated by the deaths of people like Terri Schiavo in 2005 and, for those who may remember her, Karen Carpenter, the famous singer who lost her battle with bulimia and anorexia in 1983 at the age of 33.

Few people realize the devastating impact that purging—vomiting, and/or abuse of laxatives, diuretics, enemas, or diet pills—has on the body. That's because much of the physical damage from bulimia happens internally. Besides the damage to the stomach, esophagus, and mouth as the stomach contents pass through and irritate these body regions, purging can also harm the respiratory system, cardiovascular system, metabolism, and immune system. Externally, bulimia's effects can be seen in the skin, hair, and nails, although these signs usually go unnoticed or are attributed to other causes. This failure to identify the physical signs of bulimia is part of the diagnostic dilemma.

Diagnostic Dilemma

In the doctor's office as well as out, bulimia remains a clandestine disease. Because bulimics typically deny they have a problem if and when questioned, and because no single diagnostic laboratory test can detect the disorder, bulimia often goes undiagnosed until the bulimic asks for or is convinced to seek help, or the condition is brought to the attention of a physician. In some cases, bulimia is discovered serendipitously as part of an examination or treatment for another condition or illness. Such was the case for Roxie, a nineteen-year-old college student who passed out while riding her bicycle. She broke her arm in the fall, and while she was in the hospital, lab tests revealed that her electrolytes were dangerously low. The emergency room doctor became suspicious, and after subsequent work-up and questioning, Roxie admitted that she was bulimic.

In my own practice, we generally see two types of bulimic patients: those who know they are bulimic and those who do not. At this point in my examination, I pause and ask my assistant to step around the corner for a moment. I then ask the patient if it is alright and if they would mind if I ask them questions as part of my observations and understanding of their dental condition. The patient usually is open at this time and I proceed to ask about the lack of enamel on the backs of their teeth or the swollen glands they present with. I then tell them I've seen it before and it usually is caused by an eating disorder. I stop there and gauge the impact and effect.

Body language tells a lot whether the patient is receptive to my pursuing the topic further or not. As a health care professional, a negative response does not, however, give me permission to ignore the problem and only treat her dental needs. Her overall condition will not improve without her acknowledging the evidence of the disease. As a dentist, I want to restore her entire mouth, her entire oral health, and create a beautiful smile that improves her self-esteem every time she flashes it.

Physicians who suspect a patient is dehydrated or has an electrolyte imbalance caused by vomiting, as in Roxie's case, can order a chemical panel and look for hypokalemia (abnormally low potassium levels), increased BUN (blood urea nitrogen; a test of kidney function), and electrolyte imbalance (see box). Basal serum prolactin levels also may be elevated. If a physician suspects an individuals has been using ipecac (a syrup used to induce vomiting), he or she may order a test for emetine, an ingredient and byproduct of ipecac.

Physicians can also do a more thorough evaluation and look for other indications of bingeing and purging activity, including:

- Seizures
- Arrhythmia resulting from hypokalemia, which can lead to cardiac arrest and cardiac rupture; cardiomyopathy secondary to ipecac use
- Aspiration of stomach contents into the lungs, pneumomediastinum
- Rupture of the esophagus, esophagitis, delayed gastric emptying, pancreatitis
- Muscle weakness secondary to ipecac abuse and potassium deficiency, tetany
- Impaired renal function
- Skin problems, hair loss, nail abnormalities (see below)

Electrolyte Imbalance

Electrolytes are a combination of minerals that must remain in balance for the body to function properly. An electrolyte imbalance can be caused by self-induced vomiting, laxative and/or diuretic abuse, dehydration, or malnutrition, and is a common problem among bulimics. A list of electrolytes and signs and symptoms associated with a deficiency is below:

- Calcium: muscle cramps, fragile bones, insomnia, leg and arm numbness
- Magnesium: anxiety, confusion decreased body temperature and blood pressure, muscle aches, noise sensitivity, rapid pulse
- Phosphorus: bone pain, dental problems, fatigue, heart and kidney problems, irregular breathing, loss of appetite
- Potassium: chronic thirst, decreased blood pressure, muscle cramps, skin irritation
- Sodium: confusion, cramps, eye disturbances, fatigue, loss of appetite, weakness, vomiting

Matters of the Heart

Most bulimics know that purging damages the esophagus; most experience tears and strain from regular vomiting sessions. Most, however, are surprised to learn that vomiting places the most stress on the heart muscle and can do far more damage than to the esophagus.

"Once I learned how much damage I was doing to my body by vomiting several times a day, I got really scared," says Alicia, a twenty-year-old college sophomore. "At first I thought some of what I was hearing and reading was hype, but then I met Chris, and she really scared me." Chris is a twenty-four-year-old doctoral candidate who had to take a leave from her studies because of the severity of her bulimia. Alicia met her through a mutual friend who was trying to help Alicia escape the clutches of bulimia. "When Chris had a heart attack at 24," says Alicia, "she had been purging for three years, and so had I. The reality of that fact hit home for me. I didn't want to be next."

Chris's case is just one example of the cardiovascular consequences purging can have. Chronic vomiting often leads to dehydration, malnutrition, and an imbalance in electrolyte levels (see box). Use of syrup of ipecac to induce vomiting can also result in irregular heart rhythms and heart muscle disorders, which can be deadly. Low blood pressure and fainting also can occur.

Gastrointestinal Damage

When people consider the physical damage caused by bulimia, conditions associated with the impact of vomiting on the gastrointestinal tract is usually what comes to mind. Because the stomach contents contain potent acids, bringing those contents up through the esophagus (the tube that connects the mouth and stomach) and into the mouth can severely irritate the lining of the esophagus and cause bleeding and pain, a condition known as esophagitis. If the vomiting is especially violent and/or continues over a period of time, scarring can build up in the esophagus and cause it to narrow, making it difficult to swallow. The physical stress of vomiting can also cause the esophagus to rupture or tear, a life-threatening condition that requires emergency surgery.

Chronic purging can cause gastritis, a condition in which the stomach lining is inflamed. In rare cases, rapid bingeing, combined with the fact that food leaves the stomach at a much slower rate, can cause the stomach to rupture, which can cause death from peritonitis.

The abuse of laxatives can also cause problems. Use of laxatives to cause diarrhea can result in long-term problems with the function of the large intestine, including chronic intestinal inflammation, which can eventually cause permanent constipation. Diuretics (water pills) cause the body to eliminate water and salt, which can result in seriously low potassium levels. Bulimics also often regularly experience other gastrointestinal problems, including constipation, irregular bowel movements, bloating, diarrhea, abdominal cramping, and ulcers.

Musculoskeletal System

A very dangerous habit among some bulimics is the use of ipecac syrup, which is used to induce vomiting and which has been linked to deaths among people with eating disorders. Ipecac contains an ingredient called emetine, which can accumulate in the tissues over time, whether the syrup is taken in large or small doses, and cause muscle weakness and damage throughout the body, including heart muscle.

Self-induced vomiting and overuse of laxatives and/or diuretics can also lead to high alkali levels in the blood and body tissues, which can cause muscle weakness, fatigue, and constipation. Another side effect of bingeing and purging is loss of bone density and osteoporosis due to depletion of calcium, magnesium, and other essential nutrients for healthy bones. This risk is especially critical in women who engage in both bulimic and anorexic activities, and who have amenorrhea (cessation of the menstrual cycle).

Respiratory Damage

Sometimes self-induced vomiting causes the stomach contents—food particles, bacteria, and gastric acids—to be aspirated into the sinus cavities or the lungs, where they can cause irritation and pneumonia (aspiration pneumonia).

Chronic vomiting can also damage the vocal cords. Singer Katharine McPhee, the twenty-two-year-old "American Idol" runner-up in June 2006, revealed to the press in that same month that she had suffered with bulimia for years but had sought help before the competition when she realized that all the vomiting was damaging her vocal cords. If she wanted a chance at a career in singing, she said, she knew she had to stop the bulimia, so she enrolled in an eating disorder facility. Within a few months she was realizing her dream and was beating bulimia.

Although rare, some bulimics have inadvertently blocked their airway when they used a foreign object to induce vomiting. Some of these incidents, a few of which have been reported in medical journals, have been both life-threatening and life-saving. While bulimics risk suffocation and death if they swallow an object such as a toothbrush, fork, or spoon, these medical emergencies can also bring attention to a previously unrecognized eating disorder and prompt the bulimic and/or her loved ones to take action.

Kidney Damage

The kidneys remove toxins from the body, regulate acid concentrations, and maintain water balance. Chronic vomiting and/or abuse of laxatives or diuretics, however, can cause a significant loss of fluids and electrolytes (see box), resulting in dehydration and low potassium levels, and ultimately kidney stones or even kidney failure.

More than Skin Deep

The impact of bulimia on the skin, hair, and nails can vary, depending on the severity of the disease. Perhaps the most characteristic skin sign is the presence of calluses on the knuckles. Known as Russell's sign, these form on the back of some patients' hands from repeatedly placing their fist in their mouth to help them vomit. Some bulimics avoid developing calluses by using items such as toothbrushes, spoons, and pencils to help induce vomiting, all of which can be very dangerous and result in physical harm.

Dry skin (xerosis), brittle nails, and fragile, split-end hair are also common indications of bingeing and purging and are the result of dehydration and/or malnutrition. Ginny had another telltale sign: red eyes. Six years of bingeing and purging had left this twenty-six-year-old gift shop manager with broken blood vessels in her eyes from daily vomiting, sometimes two to three times a day. "I used to tell people that I had allergies and that my eyes were red and itchy from pollen and dust," she says. "I was self-conscious about my eyes, so I wore dark glasses a lot." Another skin sign of bulimia is associated with excessive use of laxatives. Many over-the-counter laxatives contain phenolphthalein, which can cause hyperpigmentation (gray or brown spots) or sores in the skin.

An Italian study reports that certain dermatological signs are clues to the presence of bulimia and that astute dermatologists should be able to detect the disease. Some of those clues include lanugo (fine hair that appears on the face, back, and arms, which is the body's attempt to retain body heat), excessive hair loss, hyperpigmentation, slower wound healing, petechiae (pinpoint sized hemorrhages of the skin), edema, livedo reticularis (bluish mottling of the skin), paronychia (type of infection around the nail), generalized pruiritus (itching), and pellagra, among others.

Dental Problems

As I have mentioned, dentists are in a unique position to detect bulimia. One of the classic signs is the loss of enamel and dentin, which usually occurs on the upper, front inside surfaces of the teeth. When the back teeth are affected, some of the biting surfaces are worn away, making these teeth at high risk of decay and infection of the nerves inside the teeth. These signs of wear generally appear after the individual has been purging for about two years, but this is only a general figure, as it depends on how often purging occurs and whether the individual is practicing good dental hygiene.

Other signs of bulimia that dentists can see are parotid gland swelling, dry mouth, and gum inflammation or trauma. I discuss these signs and others in chapter 4, and in chapter 7 I talk about the types of treatments that are needed to restore a bulimic's oral health and smile.

Self-Harm

About 25 percent of people who have an eating disorder practice self-injury or self-harm. If you have never encountered this behavior before, it may be hard to understand how or why people would intentionally cause themselves pain. First, let's look at what self-harm means.

Disordered eating behaviors such as bingeing, purging, and starving certainly are examples of self-harm. However, in a broader sense, self-harm (a.k.a. self-abuse, self-inflicted violence, self-mutilation, self-injury) refers to actions such as cutting oneself with razors or knives, burning with cigarettes or matches, hair pulling, picking the skin until it bleeds, branding, self-poisoning, and hitting a part of the body repeatedly. The most common places self-harming individuals inflict their injuries are the wrists, inner thighs, and upper arms, places where they have easy access but that can easily be hidden from others with clothing. Bulimics who self-harm are very secretive about their behavior and experience much guilt and shame about it.

Just as bingeing and purging are dysfunctional actions bulimics perform to help them cope with deep emotional pain, so, too, are self-harm behaviors such as cutting and burning. Because bulimics cannot control their emotional pain, they engage in pain that they can control.

"When I burn myself, it's pain I can control," says Titus, an eighteen-year-old college student who has been a bulimic for two years and self-harming for about six months. "It's weird, but the burning pain is better than all the other pain. It gets my mind off the stuff I can't control, the thoughts that seem to take over my mind. Sometimes I actually feel numb. I don't even feel the cigarette burn until later."

But self-injury is a lose-lose situation. Any "relief" bulimics get from injuring themselves is only temporary, because the reason they hurt emotionally has not been addressed. Instead, they are left with physical pain and scars as well as the returning, relentless emotional pain that drove them to harm themselves in the first place. Titus admits that self-injury is "almost addictive. I get kind of a high from it sometimes." This statement follows the commonly held belief that for some people, self-injury releases endorphins, the body's natural painkillers, which causes them to experience an almost pleasant feeling from their self-abuse.

The pleasant feeling is short-lived, however, and the emotional pain returns, eventually prompting self-harm again. Greta confessed that she was afraid if anyone found out she was cutting herself, they would "lock me up in a psych ward." This nineteen-year-old receptionist had kept her bulimia and self-harm a secret for nearly two years before she was confronted by her best friend and was convinced to get help. "My girlfriend saw the scars on my thighs one day, and she got very upset," says Greta. "She knew right away what was going on, because she had a cousin who had done something similar. I denied it at first, but she didn't give up. I was in a treatment facility for a while, and I've been out for nearly a year. Sometimes when I'm under a lot of stress I still think about cutting myself, but I don't do it. It's still hard, but I have a therapist and we talk about it, and I have people who care."

Most people who intentionally harm themselves are, like Greta, afraid to ask for help because they feel they are "crazy" and will be committed to a mental hospital. However, people who self-harm are typically sane individuals who are simply caught in a cycle that includes an ill-chosen coping mechanism. Once they realize they are not alone and can let go of the secret and get help, they can learn new, healthy ways to cope with their emotional pain.

BOTTOM LINE

The physical impact of bingeing and purging on the bulimic often seems inconsequential in the beginning of the disease, but the effects of chronic abuse accumulate, resulting in signs and symptoms that can affect every system in the body. Combine this insidious damage with the relentless emotional burdens associated with the disease, and it becomes easy to see how bulimia can be an all-consuming illness. If your loved one has bulimia, I hope you have a new understanding and appreciation of the struggles he or she lives with and that you come away from this chapter with a new resolve to help a bulimic restore his or her life.

CHAPTER 4

BULIMIA IS A DENTAL DISEASE

As a dentist, I am in a unique position to help individuals who are struggling with bulimia or purging disorder. I share this distinction with all of my colleagues who practice dentistry, as well as dental hygienists and dental assistants. The reason we share this responsibility is that these eating disorders, which are typically difficult to detect, manifest themselves quite distinctly in the mouth, and we have a front row seat to what unfolds there.

In fact, sometimes I don't even need to say the magic words "Open wide, please" to know something is amiss. I've been known to spot a bulimic from across a crowded room, and the reason is that once the dental damage becomes apparent, bulimics typically try to hide their teeth in a variety of ways, the most obvious being covering their mouth whenever they smile, laugh, or otherwise open their mouth so that their teeth show. Bulimics who have dental problems may look down when speaking or mumble because they are trying to hide their teeth. If they used to have a wide, open-mouth smile, they will switch to a closed-mouth smile.

Behind the closed and hand-covered lips is a person whose mouth is in severe stress: gums, teeth, tongue, palate, and throat that are suffering the damaging consequences of chronic vomiting. In this chapter I discuss the physical impact bulimia and purging disorder have on the oral health of individuals who have these eating disorders and share the stories of several patients who "turned the corner"—admitted that they have an eating disorder and then sought help to correct it before they moved on to the restorative dental work that is much more than cosmetic; it serves to heal the psyche and restore the emotional health of patients as well.

ROLE OF THE DENTIST AND DENTAL TEAM

As a dentist, I have an obligation to be concerned not just about my patients' oral health, but their overall health as well. This obligation extends to other dental personnel as well, including dental hygienists and dental assistants, who should talk to their team leader about any concerns or suspicions they have about patients with signs of bulimia, purging, or other eating disorders.

According to Colgate Oral Pharmaceuticals and the Institute of Dental Research, 28 percent of cases of bulimia are first diagnosed during a dental examination. There are two ways to look at this statistic. On the one hand, it's a fairly high percentage for a health profession that is not specially poised to deal with eating disorders. Traditionally, people think of general practitioners, gastroenterologists, or psychiatrists as the health professionals who are most likely to deal with these conditions. On the other hand, when you consider that dental professionals are usually the first ones who have access to the part of the body that can most reveal the secret of this disease, then the percentage is probably low.

If there are clear signs that a patient has bulimia or purging disorder, dentists should confront the individual in a gentle, firm, and compassionate way. In chapter 5, I discuss in depth how friends and family members can do an intervention with their loved one. Because a dentist typically has a different type of relationship with a bulimic patient, a slightly different approach should be tried. That's why in chapter 7; I explain in detail how my staff and I approach patients with bulimia. It's an approach I've had much success with, and I hope it will encourage you to seek help.

Abrasion or Erosion? Impact of Vomiting on the Teeth

Although bulimia leaves some very distinctive signs of erosion on the teeth and mouth, it's important to make several distinctions: between abrasion and erosion; between dental erosion and other types of tooth loss; and between the erosion caused by bulimia and other types of erosion. In fact, about 18 percent of adults with dental erosion can trace the wear to another cause, such as acid reflux disease.

Abrasion is the mechanical wearing away of enamel and other hard tooth structures by external substances; the most common examples include heavy toothbrushing and bruxism (teeth grinding). It's usually easy to identify the cause of abrasion, as there are patterns that show on the teeth. Heavy toothbrushing, for example, will leave a specific pattern of wear—sharp, angular—that dentists can see.

Erosion is the nonbacterial chemical dissolution of hard tooth surfaces. Teeth affected by erosion typically appear smooth and/or spoon-shaped. Situations that cause tooth erosion, and the percentages for each, are:

- 43% related to upper gastrointestinal disorder and an acid diet
- 25% related to upper gastrointestinal disorder
- 24% related to consumption of an acid-rich diet
- 6% related to habitual vomiting associated with bulimia or purging disorder
- 2% have an unknown cause

Dental erosion, regardless of the cause, is also commonly associated with teeth sensitivity to cold and heat; abrasion rarely causes this symptom.

An astute dentist can distinguish between erosion caused by bulimic vomiting and that caused by gastric reflux or an acid-rich diet, such as sucking on oranges or lemons or hard candies. Thus, a patient may tell me she isn't vomiting and is just sucking on a lot of lemons, but her teeth tell me a different story. It's really true: you can't hide bulimia from a dentist because the teeth tell the truth, regardless of what the patient says. And here's why.

The recurring vomiting of bulimia produces a pattern of erosion sometimes called perimylolysis. Erosion is first evident on the back sides of the upper central and lateral incisors (the upper four middle teeth). As the backs of these teeth wear away, the edges become thinner and thinner, which makes them very easy to chip and crack. Over time and as the disease progresses, erosion becomes evident on the following tooth surfaces, generally appearing in this order: back surfaces of the upper molars, back surfaces of the upper cuspids, biting surfaces of the upper molars, back surfaces of the upper bicuspids, biting surfaces of the upper bicuspids. This pattern of erosion differs from other patterns and so is easy for dentists to distinguish from other causes of erosion.

For example, people who eat a great deal of citrus fruit, who habitually suck on hard candies (especially those with citric acid), or who consumed a lot of soft drinks, fruit juices, or wine can experience erosion of the facial surfaces of the maxillary anterior (upper front) teeth. (As an aside, an occupational hazard of wine tasters is erosion of tooth enamel, especially since part of their job is to swish the wine in their mouth.) This pattern differs from that seen in bulimia.

Similarly, in people who have regurgitation of stomach acid related to a hiatal hernia or gastric reflux disease, the biting surfaces and backs of the upper molars, but not the anterior teeth, are affected by erosion. The lower molars usually are not affected because the tongue naturally curves to protect those teeth.

On a sad note, however, tooth erosion associated with bulimia or purging disorder usually becomes evident within three years of the start of bulimic episodes, although not every bulimic experiences significant erosion. It's also interesting that the amount of erosion is not tightly correlated with the number of times someone vomits per day or per week, but it is associated with the duration of habitual vomiting.

Impact of Purging on the Teeth

Frequent, long-term vomiting can cause many changes in the mouth that can quickly become obvious to dental personnel (see accompanying box). One of the first clear signs that someone has bulimia is erosion on the back of the upper front teeth. This occurs because when a person throws up, the digested food, which contains hydrochloric acid and other stomach acids, is forced against the backs of the upper front teeth. The acids eat away at the tooth enamel, and the loss of enamel causes the teeth to look yellow because the underlying dentin (tooth structure) is yellow. On average, it takes about three years before tooth erosion becomes obvious, although some bulimics do not notice significant erosion for several years beyond that point. The usual treatment at this stage of tooth erosion is crowns, which I discuss in chapter 7.

Dental Problems Associated with Purging (Vomiting)
Cavities (dental caries)
Tooth erosion
Gum and mouth pain
Dry mouth
Dry, cracked, sore lips
Chronic sore throat
Inflamed esophagus
Hoarseness
Small hemorrhages in the roof of the mouth
Decreased production and secretion of saliva
Enlargement of the parotid glands
Increased periodontal disease
Swallowing problems
Problems with jaw alignment, bite, and other orthodontic abnormalities

As bulimia progresses, the enamel continues to dissolve, and if the teeth are not treated the exposed dentin is susceptible to the development of cavities. Although fillings can help, they cannot completely protect the teeth against the chronic exposure to stomach acids. If the bulimic continues to vomit and aggressive treatment is not started (e.g., crowns or porcelain-laminated veneers), the teeth will continue to decay and die. Many patients are so afraid to see a dentist that they delay making an appointment until they reach this point, when they are in pain, their teeth are highly sensitive to temperature, their gums are inflamed (gingivitis), and they realize they need help quickly. At this stage of the damage, the only course that can save the teeth is root canal therapy followed by crowns to protect what remains of each affected tooth.

If the erosion is severe enough, it can alter the way the upper and lower teeth come together and make it difficult or painful to chew. In some bulimics, the stomach acids also affect the backs of the upper molar teeth, which then suffer the same fate as the front upper teeth unless vomiting is stopped and the teeth are treated.

For some bulimics, the damage to their teeth is beyond repair, and tragically they lose most or all of their teeth. Bridgette had suffered with bulimia for nearly half her life and had become an expert on hiding it from everyone she knew, including her boyfriend of five years. She started having dental problems in her mid-twenties and needed crowns on her top front teeth. She had this work done with one dentist. Then she developed gingivitis and began having problems with her bottom teeth, so she switched to another dentist. After a series of five root canals and several more crowns, which she got from two other different dentists, she began to lose teeth. She got a bridge, but over time the anchoring teeth also began to decay, and she lost them as well. By age thirty-five, she had reached the point of no return: the few teeth that remained needed to be pulled, and she needed dentures.

"I cried for a month," she says, recalling those times as "emotionally devastating." Now, at thirty-nine, she looks back and shakes her head. "I remember thinking, 'I'm only thirty-five and I have no teeth.' My grandmother still had her teeth, yet here I was having to wear dentures. I could have saved my teeth if I had just stopped the vomiting, but I couldn't ask for help. And none of the dentists I went to, except the last one, ever mentioned bulimia or an eating disorder. All of them did ask me about my family dental history, and I always said that terrible teeth ran in the family. I told one dentist that I had gastric reflux disease; I told another one that I ate oranges and lemons every day. I told all of them that I was only going to be in town for a few months, that I was being relocated out of state.

"Basically I kept running from dentist to dentist and lying to all of them. But it caught up with me, and the dentist that pulled my teeth and did my dentures did ask me if I was vomiting. I remember I burst into tears. He took care of my teeth right away because I was in such bad shape, but he also put me in contact with an eating disorder program. It's too bad I had to lose my teeth before I got help, but I'm grateful to him for helping me change my life."

Impact of Purging on the Mouth and Throat

The teeth are not the only structures in the mouth that suffer from chronic vomiting. In fact, even before the teeth show signs of erosion, evidence of bulimia may show up in the neck. "I looked like I had the mumps," says Kim, who had been purging for about four years. "I didn't know what was wrong; I even thought I had cancer. I didn't realize that my salivary glands were swollen." The salivary glands that typically swell in bulimics are the parotids, which are located at the corner of the lower jaw on the back lower sides of the face, although the submaxillary glands (located in the inner side of the lower jaw) may also be involved. These glands produce saliva that moisten your food while you chew, and are also the glands that swell if you get the mumps. The swelling makes you look like your jowls are enlarged. Although the swelling is soft and pliable in the beginning, with continued vomiting the swelling becomes hard and permanent over time.

Many bulimics force themselves to vomit by pushing two fingers of their hand down their throat. This typically causes sores or scars to form on the back of the hand that is used. Some people, however, occasionally or routinely use other objects, such as toothbrushes, spoons, tongue depressors, or forks to induce vomiting, which is dangerous and can cause lacerations and/or bruising of the throat.

Occasionally, a bulimic's bite (the way their teeth mesh together) changes because routinely pushing a hand into the mouth can cause the jaw joints to shift. The result is chronic temporomandibular joint (TMJ/TMD) related facial pain. Other oral problems associated with bulimia include a dry, sore mouth, burning tongue, chronic sore throat, and small hemorrhages of the palate caused by scratches from fingernails or other objects when the patient induces vomiting.

A Step in the Right Direction

The deterioration and loss of their smile is very disturbing for many bulimics and those with purging disorder, and fear about whether they will ever be able to smile with confidence—and without pain—is something I see and hear often in my practice. Fortunately, for those who are willing to accept personal responsibility and seek treatment to rid themselves of their eating disorder, restoration of their shining smile and repair of other oral health issues can be achieved. The actual degree of help required is highly individual and depends on the extent of the damage, as I discuss in chapter 7.

Steps to restore your smile and your oral health can only begin in earnest once you pursue treatment and your bulimia or purging disorder is under control. Essentially, it is a waste of time, money, and energy to do extensive restorative dental work while you are actively purging.

But that does not mean you can't take some steps to be "good to your mouth" as you begin treatment for your eating disorder and during the early stages of your recovery, until you reach a point where purging is under control and focused dental restoration can begin. My colleagues and I typically offer the following guidelines for these patients.

- DO NOT brush your teeth after vomiting, because stomach acid weakens the enamel and brushing can cause additional erosion of your teeth. It can be helpful to brush immediately before vomiting, however.
- You can also rinse your mouth with mouthwash that contains 0.05 percent fluoride. Fluoride helps strengthen teeth.
- When you do brush, use a soft brush and a toothpaste that contains fluoride.
- To help dry mouth, drink water to keep your mouth moist. If you have reduced saliva production, you can use a saliva replacement, which your dentist can prescribe, or chew sugar-free gum.
- If your teeth are severely damaged and you are in treatment for bulimia, your dentist may be able to prescribe an appliance that covers your teeth and protects them from damaging stomach acids.
- As a rule, avoid acid foods and beverages (e.g., citrus fruits and juices, tomatoes, vinegar, pickled foods)
- Reduce your intake of alcohol, including ciders, mixers, and wine
- Floss every day

BOTTOM LINE

There is no question that chronic vomiting causes a great deal of damage to the teeth, mouth, and throat. Not only do bulimics have to deal with the resulting physical pain and discomfort, but also the emotional turmoil associated with losing their smile. The good news is that with treatment—first addressing the emotional issues associated with bulimia and then restorative dental work—the smiles return. In the next section I talk about how to begin and carry through the treatment process, along with an entire chapter on the type of dental work that can be done to help bulimics learn to smile again.

CHAPTER 5

STEP 1:
FACE-TO-FACE WITH BULIMIA

"I'm in recovery from bulimia today, and lucky to be alive, because two years ago someone had the courage to say to me, 'I think you have some problems with food and I want to help you overcome them, because I love you and I know you're worth it.'" Twenty-eight-year-old Nadine, sitting in a Seattle Starbucks, wipes a few tears from her eyes and smiles. "I still get emotional when I think about it, because I wanted help yet I was too ashamed and too embarrassed to ask for it. I was bingeing and purging two or three times a day, I was depressed, and I was afraid to go out. I worked at home as a freelance graphic artist, and I only had to visit clients a few times a week, so I was alone a lot. I couldn't stop bingeing and purging. I really think I would have died if Kyle hadn't stepped in."

Nadine was fortunate that her best friend, Kyle, took the initiative and confronted her with her suspicions. Before she spoke with Nadine, Kyle had done her homework: she read books and articles about bulimia, searched the internet for the latest studies and articles offered by various organizations, and then decided she had enough information to take matters into her own hands.

"I knew I needed to make Nadine feel safe and to let her know that I love her and that she is a big part of my life," says Kyle. "I admit I was a little apprehensive about confronting her, but I'm so glad I did. Just look at her today!"

Most people who have an eating disorder do not seek treatment on their own, but they typically will get help if they are prompted and supported by a partner, parent, friend, or doctor. In this chapter, I talk about how you can offer the impetus and support to a loved one so he or she will feel safe. For bulimics, part of feeling safe is being able to put aside at least some of their shame, guilt, and fear in order to come face-to-face with their disease, admit they need help, and then accept that help from someone they trust.

Because most of the people who first develop bulimia do so during their preteen or teen years, parents, as well as older siblings, other family members, and school officials, are very often in a position to notice signs and symptoms of an eating disorder and to take appropriate action. Yet all too often this doesn't happen for various reasons. Concerned family and others often don't know what signs to look for, or the indications may be too subtle, or they may suspect something is wrong but don't know how to approach the person. And because bulimia is usually not "in your face," it can be easy to deny or ignore. Unfortunately, those who suffer with the disease cannot ignore it or the toll it takes on the body.

As a dentist I have reached out to individuals who sat in my office with the telltale signs of bulimia. Over the years I've been fortunate to have been able to assist most of them in getting the treatment help they needed, and then had the privilege of restoring their oral health and smiles when they were ready for that step. For a detailed explanation of how I personally handle bulimic patients in my office, from the moment they first come in either admitting or denying the disease, until they walk out with a restored smile, see chapter 7.

This chapter, however, is about you. Here I talk about how you can come face-to-face with bulimia; whether you are (1) someone who has the disease; or (2) a concerned parent, spouse, friend, family member, dentist, or other health professional who suspects or recognizes that there is a problem and who wants to help. Drawing upon the insight from women who have bulimia and some of their loved ones, I discuss how to recognize if there is a problem (including checklists to help identify bulimia and purging disorder), various ways to approach the subject of bulimia with affected individuals, where to turn for help, and how to find a doctor and/or treatment facility.

WHEN TO SEEK HELP

There is only one time to seek help when someone has bulimia or purging disorder: NOW. "Bingeing and purging was the center of my life for years," says Matthew, an Olympic hopeful in Greco-Roman wrestling. "I planned my life around when and how I could binge and then vomit. Every time I vomited, I swore I would stop, that I would try to get some help and never binge and purge again. But I broke that vow again and again until one day my sister, herself a recovering bulimic, came to visit me, sat me down, and said she would do whatever it took to help me. She said she wasn't going to leave until the two of us took steps to get me into treatment. She helped me get my life back."

It's never too soon or too late to get help. If you've binged and purged a few times and think, "I can control this," get help now before the bulimia gets out of hand. If you are like Matthew and have been bingeing and purging for some time, the need to act now is even more urgent, as every bulimic episode results in more physical, emotional, and spiritual harm.

Similarly, if you suspect a loved one is bulimic, the time to prepare for an intervention is now. I talk about how to prepare for and then conduct an intervention in this chapter.

DOES MY LOVED ONE HAVE BULIMIA

"I didn't suspect anything because my daughter didn't look sick," says Arlene as she nervously fussed with the bracelet on her left wrist. "She never lost a lot of weight and she never complained about not feeling well or about not wanting to go to school. I did notice that she was withdrawing a lot from my husband and I, but I thought that was typical fifteen-year-old behavior. When she started avoiding most of her friends and acting secretive around the house and staying in her room a lot, I thought she might be involved with drugs. And in a way she was: food was her drug. I just never imagined she had bulimia."

Because people with bulimia often don't "look sick," their loved ones and friends often don't realize they have the disease or, if they do suspect or know, they usually don't realize the seriousness of the situation. If the person is both anorexic and bulimic, there may be more clues, especially if he or she has lost a great deal of weight. But in most cases of bulimia, the individual is of normal weight or even slightly overweight, and so no "warning" signs are obvious.

One important thing to remember is that bulimia is not about weight; it's about distorted, self-defeatist thinking and beliefs that lead people to practice harmful behaviors. As we've discussed, bulimics usually have low self-esteem and are often filled with self-loathing; they may say they hate themselves or that they want to die. They need help to see that they are truly valuable, caring individuals who are loved.

Recognizing and Defining Bulimia

Before early 2005, many people had never heard of Terri Schiavo. Ms. Schiavo was the young woman in Florida who lapsed into a vegetative state after she suddenly collapsed in her home in February 1990 at the age of twenty-six. Experts later revealed that her condition was the result of a dangerously low potassium level, which caused her heart to stop and blood flow to the brain to be interrupted, resulting in brain damage. The cause of her lethally low potassium level was bulimia.

No one knew Terri was bulimic until it was too late. One reason no one knew she was ill is because bulimia can be difficult to recognize. Difficult, but certainly not impossible.

Depending on your relationship with the person you suspect may have bulimia, you may be more or less able or likely to observe various physical signs of the disease. Certainly, as someone's dentist, I am not privy to the day-to-day behaviors or the psychological signs of bulimia. But I am able to get a unique look at the individual's dental picture, which literally speaks a thousand words. You, however, can use the following checklists to help you. The more "yes" answers, the greater the likelihood that he or she (or you) has bulimia.

[CHECKLIST:]
Physical and Behavioral Signs of Bulimia

Does the individual:

o   Vomit after eating? Although you may not actually witness or hear the person vomit, you may note that she regularly retreats to a bathroom immediately or soon after eating, both at home and when eating out. Hints that the individual may be vomiting include running the water in the sink or shower for a long period of time and/or flushing the toilet several times. There are also some physical signs of vomiting, listed below.

o   Engage in excessive and/or compulsive exercise? One mother said she could hear her daughter running in place in her room for hours nearly every night. Some bulimics exercise excessively only when they are unable to vomit; others use exercise along with vomiting on a regular basis.

o   Abuse laxatives, diet pills, diuretics, or drugs that induce vomiting? (See the accompany story about Patricia.) You may find a stash of these items in the house or see many empty packages in the trash.

o   Leave behind evidence that large amounts of food have been consumed? Sweets and/or other carbohydrates (e.g., cookies, doughnuts, candy, snack cakes, bread, crackers) are the foods most often used during a binge. You may find many empty food wrappers in the trash, hidden in a closet, a car, or backpack.

o   Hoard food? You may find food hidden in closets, under the seat of the car, under clothes in bureaus, under the bed. One mother found her daughter's hidden cookie supply inside a huge stuffed bear that was in her daughter's room. The stuffing had been removed and replaced by bags of cookies and marshmallows.

o   Avoid eating in front of other people? The person may regularly create or find excuses to avoid sharing meals with you or others.

o   Decline to eat out if it was an activity she once enjoyed?

o   When eating with you, does she avoid carbohydrates or avoid eating at all?

o   Seem preoccupied with counting calories and/or fat grams, reading recipes, looking at food labels, or talking about food?
o   Spend an unusual amount of money on food?
o   Hide his/her smile or mouth because of bad teeth? This is a habit I see often: the person immediately covers her mouth with a hand or another object, looks down so as to avoid showing her mouth, or tries to avoid smiling altogether. A closed-lips smile may be an indication of a serious self-image issue.
o   Have dental problems (loose, stained, broken, abscessed teeth; bleeding or swollen gums) that seem to have come on suddenly or are new?
o   Have dry skin, nails, and/or hair? This is usually the result of dehydration and/or malnutrition (see chapter 2)
o   Constantly have cold-like symptoms, such as coughing, sniffling, hoarseness, and sneezing? These are side effects of vomiting.
o   Have red eyes? This sign is usually due to blood vessels that rupture from chronic vomiting.
o   Have swollen salivary glands (especially in the neck)? Although there are also salivary glands in the mouth, those in the neck will be more obvious and may be the size of a golf ball.
o   Spend a lot of time in front of a mirror and/or checking weight?
o   Have scars or calluses on the backs of her hands from sticking her fingers down her throat to vomit? This sign actually has a name: Russell's sign
o   Drink a lot of diet soda or water? This is a tactic used to feel full as well as help one vomit easier.

NOTE: For a more intense and personal checklist, "Do I Have Bulimia?" see the appendix. This checklist contains about 100 statements and is designed to be completed by a person who thinks he or she may be bulimic.

Patricia's Story

"When I think about it now, I see not only how dangerous it was, but how irrational as well," says Patricia, a twenty-four-year-old nail technician and recovering bulimic. "I mean, I was taking large doses of laxatives, which cleaned out my bowels, but the calories from any food I allowed myself to keep down—and I was vomiting after every binge and nearly every meal—had already been absorbed by my body. So what I lost when using laxatives was fluid—and lots of important electrolytes."

Patricia was among the estimated one-third of bulimics who abuse over-the-counter as well as prescription laxatives as part of their purging activity. During her time at a treatment center, she came to understand just how dangerous her misuse of laxatives had been. Although she experienced some of the side effects of chronic laxative abuse, including bloating, stomach cramps, and dehydration, fortunately she got help before she progressed to more serious consequences, including irregular heartbeat, renal problems, electrolyte imbalances, cardiac arrhythmias, and death.

People who have abused laxatives for a prolonged time can expect to have some withdrawal symptoms for several weeks or longer, depending on how long they abused the drugs. Patricia was no exception. "I experienced some of the same symptoms I had when I was taking the laxatives, like stomach cramps and bloating," she says. "But I also had constipation, crazy mood swings, and lots of fatigue for several weeks before all the symptoms finally went away," she says.

Although Patricia didn't use diuretics (sometimes referred to as "water pills"), an estimated 10 percent of bulimics do, either alone or along with laxatives, to control their weight. Like laxatives, these drugs can decrease the amount of water in the body and result in dehydration and electrolyte (especially potassium) imbalances that may require hospitalization. People who have abused diuretics often find that they experience fluid retention even after they discontinue taking the water pills.

[CHECKLIST:]
Psychological Signs of Bulimia

People with bulimia typically experience some, many, or most of the following psychological signs of the disease. These signs are often less obvious than physical ones. But if you observe and talk with someone you suspect has bulimia and look and listen for these clues, they may become very evident and fit into a larger picture, along with physical signs of the disease. When looking for these clues, ask yourself: Are any of these feelings new or significantly more pronounced than in the past? Do these feelings seem to be persistent and/or present most or all of the times you see this person?

- Feelings of helplessness, loneliness, and isolation
- Consistent denial of hunger
- Acting secretive
- Depression, characterized by a lack of interest in things that used to be of interest (e.g., sex, friends, hobbies), sleep difficulties, change in weight (up or down)
- Black and white thinking. The person sees the world in terms of extremes: things are either good or bad, perfect or completely wrong, successful or a failure; there is no room for compromise or discussion.
- Anxiety and/or panic attacks
- Low self-esteem (may be characterized by self-deprecating remarks, such as "I'm never right," "I'm never good enough," or "I'm so stupid") and/or lack of self-confidence
- Feelings of shame and guilt
- Distorted perception of body shape and weight (makes remarks about being fat, out of proportion, looking "gross," and so on)
- Feeling out of control when around food, such as having an uncontrollable urge to eat several boxes of cookies or a dozen doughnuts
- Mood swings that may be accompanied by crying spells
- Great difficulty making even small decisions; e.g., can't decide what to wear to school, which movie to watch on television, or whether to go to the store or stay home
- Intense feeling of doom

PURGING DISORDER

As I mentioned in chapter 2, purging disorder is a condition distinct from bulimia in that individuals purge but do not binge. At one time, this type of eating disorder was classified by DSM-IV in a category known as Eating Disorder Not Otherwise Specified (EDNOS). But recent research indicates that purging disorder is not only a clinically significant and distinctive eating disorder, but that it appears to be even more prevalent than anorexia and bulimia combined. If this is true, then there are millions more people who are exposing themselves to the physical consequences and emotional turmoil of purging.

Research into the specifics of purging disorder is in its infancy, but so far it appears that because these people don't binge, they tend to purge based on what they eat rather than on how much. That is, while bulimics typically purge after eating an abnormally large amount of food, people with purging disorder may purge after eating a very small amount or something they perceive as being "wrong" to eat.

Cornelia's Story

Cornelia is an example. This thirty-one-year-old computer programmer has been purging for "about five years, ever since my son was born." After gaining nearly forty pounds with her pregnancy, Cornelia joined a weight loss club and lost thirty pounds. But the last 10 pounds wouldn't budge, and she was worried that she would gradually regain the weight she had lost. "At first I was throwing up one or two times a week," she says, "and gradually I increased it to about four or five times. That's about where I am now. Whenever I eat a normal meal, what I call a 'healthy meal,' like a salad and a piece of broiled chicken, I don't throw up. But if I splurge and eat a few cookies or a piece of cake, then I force myself to vomit. I never binge eat. I've been able to keep my weight pretty steady at 130, which is about 10 pounds more than I weighed before I had my son."

Cornelia says she doesn't consider herself to have an eating disorder, but rather a "proven diet method, a way to keep my weight down." Unfortunately, she is mistaken. As I mentioned, people who have purging disorder expose themselves to the same health-related consequences as those who have bulimia.

Identifying Purging Disorder

While bulimics can be a challenge to identify, those with purging disorder may be even more difficult, because their purging behavior is less consistent and even more elusive. If you suspect a loved one has purging disorder, you can use the checklists we've provided for bulimia. However, because purging disorder does not involve bingeing behaviors, you will need to be especially vigilant and observant to detect indications of this disorder. For example, if you are with the person when she has an opportunity to eat "forbidden" foods, such as at a birthday party or other special occasion, you can observe if she disappears to a bathroom after eating dessert. It is very likely she will eat only a very small amount of dessert, yet still feel the need to purge.

You might also pay special attention to the person's teeth. One resourceful woman named Delia says she suspected her friend Ellie was purging because she sometimes disappeared after into the restroom after eating "sinful desserts" whenever they ate at a restaurant. "I also noticed that she was being much more guarded about her mouth, looking down whenever she laughed or putting her hand near her mouth. So one day I said, 'Ellie, you've got something black stuck in your front teeth,' which wasn't true, and she immediately put her hand over her mouth. I said, 'let me see if it's gone," and she looked panicked and pulled away from me. I felt bad because I had lied, but her behavior supported my suspicions. I asked her what was wrong, and that's when she broke down and admitted her teeth looked terrible. She didn't admit to purging right then, but as we talked about her teeth, I eventually asked her if the problem was because she was purging, and she admitted it."

Delia's confrontation with her friend was Ellie's turning point: with her friend's help Ellie was able to get help for her eating disorder and eventually stop her purging behavior. Such confrontations, or interventions, can be life changing and even life saving for people with bulimia. Let's look at how interventions work.

"WE NEED TO TALK"

Confronting someone who has bulimia to encourage her or him to get help is one of the most caring, loving actions you can take: it can literally save that person's life. It also is a very sensitive matter, and one that requires careful planning on your part

One of the first things you need to do is learn all you can about bulimia. Reading this book—and reviewing the checklists—is a good start; so is referring to some of the resources listed in the appendix. Arming yourself with knowledge is important because the individual you confront will likely deny that she has an eating disorder or that she needs any help. It will help if you feel secure in your knowledge of the facts as well as treatment options. Thus, along with the results of your review of the checklists, personal observations, and general information about bulimia, you should also be prepared with a list of professionals, organizations, and groups that can be helpful.

Once you feel confident you have enough information, you can prepare to talk with the individual. Choose a time and place that is comfortable, quiet, and private; you may want to suggest the two of you go for a walk or get together for coffee or tea at your house. (Do not suggest you get together for food. You want the focus to be on her emotional needs, not the food she uses to deal with them.) If you are a parent who is confronting your teenager at home, make sure you choose a time when you will not be interrupted. You and your teen may feel more comfortable away from home; you may let him or her choose the place for your talk.

Be Prepared

"De Nial" is not a river in Egypt—it is what you can expect from the person you suspect has bulimia. Along with words of denial, be prepared to be challenged repeatedly. Individuals with bulimia and other eating disorders typically not only deny they have a problem, they will also resist your efforts to help them and will insist that whatever they are doing is okay or necessary. Naturally, this is distorted thinking, but you need to be calm, firm, and supportive. The individual may continue to deny there is a problem even after the two of you have talked about the issue several times. **Don't give up!** You are planting seeds of change, and the fact that the person is meeting with you, even if she hasn't yet taken the steps to get help, is a sign that she is listening. Continue to insist that professional help is critical.

It's also important for you to realize that any resistance and denial coming from the person you are confronting is not directed against you but against the fear of losing control, feelings of helplessness, fear of change, and fear of gaining weight.

Confrontation

Now it's time to come face-to-face. Remember: you need to be firm but supportive, nonjudgmental, and loving in your words, tone, and attitude:

- Begin by reassuring the person that you care a great deal about her and that you greatly value your relationship. In that context, explain that you are concerned about her health and well-being and that you have observed some behaviors and changes in her appearance that worry you. Be calm and emphatic and do not back down or argue if she begins to deny that anything is wrong.
- Listen carefully to what the individual has to say in reply. Do not interrupt her. This is NOT the time to offer advice or to make judgments. Your job is to listen
- Encourage her to talk about her feelings—what worries her, causes her pain. Remember that bulimia is about feelings and the misuse of food to solve emotional problems, and not about food or weight per se. Ask her how she feels about different aspects of her life, such as school, work, music, friends, and hobbies.
- Offer to help her in any way you can, and then present her with some suggestions. Do not say, "Let me know what I can do to help" because that gives her an opening to reply, "there's nothing you can do" or "I don't want help" or "I don't need help." You must take some control over the situation and present some solid options.
- Encourage her to contact you whenever she needs to talk. She needs to know that someone—you—are willing to listen to her without judging. Even if she is not ready to seek professional help at that moment, you need to let her know that you are not willing to give up.
- Make a definite appointment with her to talk again and set a goal to be reached by that next meeting. You may, for example, agree that she will talk with one of the professionals on your list or visit a treatment center. Offer to go with her to any appointments she may make. If these steps are too ambitious for the moment, she may agree to read this book or a particular article about bulimia and then tell you her feelings about it.

- Conclude your time by restating how much you value your relationship and that you want to facilitate her recovery in any way you can.
- As always, there is a list of things you **should not** say or do. I've included such a list as a sidebar ("What Not To Say Or Do").

Here is the "What Not to Say or Do" list to keep in mind when you talk to a person who has bulimia and you are offering support and information. Do not:

- Place blame or criticism or be judgmental. Telling a person that she "should know better" or is "stupid" or "sick" is not constructive. Her self-esteem is already extremely low.
- Get into long discussions about eating, dieting, weight, or food. Bulimia is not about food. Food is only the instrument bulimics use to deal with other problems.
- Oversimplify the situation. Use of phrases like "all you have to do is . . ." or "It will be easy to . . ." or "bulimia is just an addiction" trivializes the situation. Bulimia is a serious disease and should be treated as such.
- Glamorize it. Bulimia exists in a realm of mystery, but don't perpetuate it. Familiarize yourself with some of the hard facts about bulimia (as we've discussed in chapter 2) and quote them when necessary.
- Confront the person in the company of other people. This will be embarrassing and only alienate the person from you.
- Give the person advice about exercise or dieting.
- Give false hope. Telling someone "If you stop bingeing and purging, everything will be fine" is a great disservice. The bulimia is a symptom of an underlying psychological issue that needs to be addressed.
- Fight. If the person keeps denying there is a problem, remain calm. Do not raise your voice or argue; simply restate your concerns, observations, and willingness to help. If either of you becomes too emotional, suggest that you both meet again soon when emotions have settled.

After the Challenge

The first time you confront someone who has bulimia, you may not be successful in convincing him or her to get professional help. The second time may do the trick, or it may get you closer to your goal but still require a few more attempts. The important thing is that you continue to offer unconditional love and support to the individual, even though he or she may continue to deny and challenge your concern.

Binge Eating Disorder

People with binge eating disorder typically eat large amounts of food at least twice a week, usually in a very short time, but do not purge. This eating behavior is their way to avoid painful emotions and/or anxiety, yet food makes them feel out of control. Binge eaters often avoid social situations where food is served because they are afraid they will binge in public. Most people with binge eating disorder are overweight or obese and often have high blood pressure, type 2 diabetes, and/or high cholesterol.

Although we have been focusing on the dangers of purging, it's important for you to recognize binge eating behaviors as well, as some people begin with binge eating and then "graduate" to bulimia. Thus if you can identify and stop binge eating before it progresses to bulimia, you've helped prevent a potentially life-threatening disorder.

The following is a list of symptoms of binge eating disorder. The more "yes" answers you have, the greater the likelihood that someone you know (or you) has binge eating disorder.

o   Frequently eats an excessive amount of food within a short period of time (in private and/or in public)
o   Eats rapidly
o   Often eats in private or alone so as to hide his/her eating habits. When eating with other people, eats only small amounts
o   Eats until feeling uncomfortable or ill
o   Shows disgust, irritation, or self-loathing after overeating
o   Does not purge by vomiting, exercising vigorously, or abusing laxatives, diuretics, and/or diet pills
o   Is usually sedentary

HOW TO START A DIALOGUE

Before you confront the individual who has bulimia, you may find it helpful to rehearse what you plan to say and how the other person might respond or challenge you. One mother who is a paralegal noted that this type of preparation is similar to how a lawyer prepares a witness to take the stand.

The following sample script for an intervention can help you understand how an intervention may proceed and help prepare you for denials, rebuttals, and other comments or challenges the person you are confronting may make. In this sample, you will notice that the parent doesn't mention the words "eating disorder" or "bulimia" during the first few exchanges. You may or may not feel comfortable using these words in your opening, depending on your relationship with the person and whether you think introducing the words too soon in the conversation may scare the individual even further. This sample below is between a parent and child, but if the person you are talking to is someone else—a spouse, friend, co-worker, or other adult—you can use it as a model and make adjustments to fit your own situation. For example, you may want to talk about some of the physical impact of bulimia by asking the individual if she has been experiencing any pain, lightheadedness, or other symptoms. The person with bulimia may be reluctant to admit she/he has any of these problems and be relieved that you asked.

Sample Intervention

Parent: Lately I've been very worried about you, and so I'd like to share some of my concerns with you now. I have noticed that [describe what you have observed, both physical and psychological. When you describe psychological signs, use phrases like "you seem to be sad" or "you appear to be _____" to convey that these are your observations and not labels you are placing on the person.]

Child: I'm fine. There's nothing wrong. [Or, "It's none of your business," "Everything is fine," or "Leave me alone."]

Parent: Perhaps you can tell me why you think everything is alright, because it appears we don't see this situation in the same way. [Or, "It isn't possible for me to leave you alone or ignore what I am seeing because I care about you. Perhaps you can explain why I shouldn't worry about you."]

Child: I don't want to talk about it. [Or, "There's nothing to talk about. I'm okay."]

Parent: I am concerned because I believe your health is at risk. Since you and I appear to see this situation differently, perhaps we need to have a third party, a professional, help us understand it better and help us decide if we need to do anything about it.

Child: I don't need to see anybody because nothing's wrong. [Or, "I'm not going to talk to a stupid doctor," or "I can take care of everything myself."]

Parent: I want you to know that I'm saying these things because I care about you and because I'm frightened for you. It's very natural to feel scared when you don't understand something or when you feel out of control. Having an eating disorder makes you feel out of control, but it doesn't have to be that way. Many people don't understand eating disorders and so they say stupid or wrong things about them, like you can never get better or that you're crazy. But these things are not true. Do you understand that?

Child: I know there's nothing wrong with me. I just don't want to be fat so I'm trying to keep my weight down. I wish you'd leave me alone.

Parent: Most people think eating disorders are about food and weight and being fat. I used to think that was true, too. But bulimia is actually a technique people use to help them cope with their emotions and stress and to help them take control of food and their lives. The thing is, bulimia is about being out of control with food. So if you're out of control with food, you are probably feeling out of control in other parts of your life as well. I'd like to help you get a better handle on those things in your life that seem of your control so you don't have to do such extreme things in order to lose weight.

Child: I don't think I have a problem, but if I did, how do I know things will get better if I get help? Can you guarantee that?

Parent: Overcoming an eating disorder can be a challenge, but you are a strong, intelligent, and capable person, and I believe you can do it. And I will be with you all the way, supporting and helping you in any way I can. We can find a program that will allow you to continue on with your life and your activities as much as possible, without making too many changes. I promise we will work together with a professional to make this process as smooth as possible.

Child: I don't want to leave school (college). It's too important to me.

Parent: I certainly can understand that, and I want you to be able to continue with your education. But even if you needed to take a little time off, perhaps one semester, you may be able to keep up with your work off-campus. But what's most important is for you to beat this eating disorder so you can regain control of your life.

Child: I have to think about it for a while. I don't want to talk about it any more right now.

Parent: I can appreciate your wanting to think about it, but the longer you allow this eating disorder to take control of you, the more you are harming your body and the harder it will be to shake it. Let's make a compromise: I'm willing to wait a week if you can take that week to consider what we've talked about today and to try to make any changes on your own. Then one week from today we will get together and talk about it again and make some firm plans at that time. Can you promise to do that?

Child: I guess that sounds okay. But I still don't think I need help.

Parent: If someone you cared a great deal about was doing something harmful or dangerous, wouldn't you want to help that person or bring the situation to his or her attention? ("If _____ [a best friend] were involved in something dangerous, wouldn't you want to help her and protect her?") That's what I'm doing here.

Child: I don't think you need to protect me, because nothing's wrong with me. Why do you want to change me? Aren't I good enough the way I am?

Parent: Of course you are good enough. But an eating disorder is not who you are, it is not part of your identity. Having an eating disorder prevents you from being all you can be, the loving, caring person that you are, because it takes control of you. I just want to help you rid yourself of this "thing" that is taking control of you. So we agree that you will think about our discussion and be prepared to take some steps next week when we talk again.

CAN BULIMIA BE PREVENTED?

As I mentioned in chapter 2, parents do not **cause** their child's eating disorder, but they do play a part in forming a child's ideas and perspectives about food, weight, body image, and self-esteem. Therefore, the types of messages that parents (and other authority figures, such as other adult family members, coaches, and teachers) pass along to children about these issues can have an impact on any future development of an eating disorder.

If you are the parent, you can evaluate your own behaviors and thoughts about food, weight, and body image by answering the following questions. Do you believe or give the impression that:

- You must be thin to be happy and successful
- Heavy people are stupid, unattractive, and/or unworthy of love
- Food is fattening
- Enjoying food is wrong or "sinful"
- All fat is unhealthy
- Fasting, skipping meals, and dieting are healthy ways to keep your weight under control
- The more exercise you do, the thinner you can be

If you answer "yes" to any of these statements, all of which are false, then you may be unintentionally giving out messages that can fuel bulimia or another eating disorder.

Actions speak louder than words, and so if you are a parent, one way for you to teach your child healthy eating habits and healthy ideas about weight, body image, and him/herself as an individual is through example. Ask yourself the following questions: Do you

- Have a kitchen that is stocked with healthy foods?
- Make sure your child gets three nutritious meals per day
- Eat as many meals with your child (and other family members) as possible
- Serve a variety of foods
- Make sure meal times are calm and stress-free
- Avoid making negative remarks about eating, weight, or body image in front of your child. These can be remarks about yourself or other family members.
- Emphasize good nutrition rather than the concept of 'dieting' as the best way for good health
- Teach your child that the body and brain require nutritious food to operate at their best
- Intervene if your child is self-deprecating. Remarks such as "I'm stupid," "I'm always wrong," and "I can't do anything right" should be countered with positive statements from you, such as "Everyone makes mistakes. It's just important to learn from them," and "I'm always so proud of you when you (fill in the blank)."
- Encourage your child to explore his or her own interests, not yours. Children should be encouraged to pursue activities that interest them, not ones solely to please their parents.

Practicing and projecting healthy attitudes about food, weight, and self are smart steps for everyone to follow. If you are a parent, these ideals are important for every child, not just one whom you think may have a tendency to develop an eating disorder. Remember: it doesn't matter who has an eating disorder in a family, as that person's behaviors and emotions impact everyone in the family. An eating disorder is a family affair.

WHERE TO GET HELP

Be assured, help is available. It's easy to think otherwise if you are in the throes of bulimia or if you are worried about your child or spouse or best friend who is bingeing and purging. That's why it's important to stay calm and to review the options available to you, given any special needs or limitations you may have; for example, accessibility to a treatment center (if one is needed), number of eating disorder specialists in your area, ability to travel some distance if expert help is not close at hand, and type of insurance coverage. The following tips can help you with this task.

Finding a Medical Practitioner

Whether you are looking for a physician for yourself or for a loved one, for a child, adolescent, or older individual, it's important to find a qualified individual as well as one with whom you feel confident and comfortable. The role of this professional is to do a medical assessment and to act as the doctor who oversees the treatment program. He or she should be able to refer you to appropriate therapists, nutritionists, and/or treatment facilities (if needed), although you can (and I suggest, should) investigate possibilities on your own as well. I have listed several resources in the appendix for this purpose.

When looking for such a health-care practitioner, consider someone who:

- Has experience in eating disorders, preferably a board-certified adolescent medicine practitioner if the individual with bulimia is a child or adolescent.
- Takes the time to answer your questions thoroughly
- Was referred to you by someone who used the practitioner for bulimia or another eating disorder (this isn't always possible, but can be helpful if it is)
- Doesn't rush you or seem annoyed by your questions
- Can be reached 24 hours a day
- Is willing to discuss various treatment approaches
- Seems like someone you can trust. This may be a "gut" feeling, but it is an important one.
- Is willing to give you recommendations from other patients or parents who have gone through the same experience

You should also check to see if an ethics board has ever disciplined the physician or had a license suspended or revoked. You can call your state licensing board and inquire about the license, credentials, and ethical violations of health-care providers, including therapists, in your state.

Various organizations also maintain lists of practitioners who specialize either in eating disorders and/or adolescent medicine. Information on how to contact these organizations is in the appendix.

Finding a Therapist

In most cases of bulimia, the first place to turn once any serious medical conditions have been ruled out is psychiatric treatment. This is the cornerstone of therapy for bulimia since the reasons for the distorted eating behaviors are emotionally based. (I discuss various types of psychiatric approaches in depth in chapter 5.) Here is where you definitely need someone who specializes in eating disorders, bulimia in particular.

One natural place to begin your search is with your primary care physician: ask him or her for referrals for eating disorders therapists. If you know someone who has had a problem similar to yours and who worked with a therapist, you can ask whether he or she would recommend the individual. You can also contact professional organizations that maintain referral lists of qualified practitioners (see Appendix). If the individual who needs therapy is an adolescent, look for a therapist or psychologist who specialists in adolescent therapy.

You should verify the credentials of any therapist you are considering, as some people call themselves therapists but do not have the proper credentials to make that claim. If you are considering psychiatrists (who are MDs and thus licensed to dispense medication), ask if they had residency training in psychiatry and are board certified in psychiatry. (Not all psychiatrists are board certified; however lack of certification does not mean a psychiatrist is not qualified to deal with eating disorders.) For psychologists, ask if they are licensed as a psychologist and if not, what license they practice under and what their specific training has been. Therapists should be questioned about the type of license, degree, and training they have.

You should also consider whether you or your loved one wants to work with a same-sex therapist or one of the opposite sex. This is an important issue for many people and it can make or break the success of the therapy experience.

Most of the questions used when considering a physician can also be used to help you choose a therapist (see above). In addition, consider the following questions:

- Does the therapist do family therapy? This may be important if you are a parent whose child is bulimic and family therapy is recommended.
- What types of therapy methods are used? I talk more about the various types of therapeutic approaches in chapter 6 and 9.
- How long are the sessions and how often are they?
- Is the therapist associated with or have visiting privileges with a specific treatment facility? This may be important if you or your loved one needs to go into treatment.
- Does the therapist accept your insurance and how are co-payments handled?

Ideally, you should talk to several therapists before you make your selection. Your first session with a therapist is for the purpose of deciding whether you can work with the individual. Allow yourself a day or two after the session to think about how the encounter went and how you felt during and after. Did you feel comfortable with the therapist? Did the therapist listen to you and seem genuinely interested in what you had to say? Do you think you can trust this therapist? Did the therapist seem open to your suggestions and comments? Did the therapist discuss how therapy works? Did you discuss or set some goals during the visit?

If you or your loved one was not comfortable with the therapist or with how the session progressed, consider another therapist. Sometimes it takes several tries to find the right expert, and working with a mental health professional who is compatible is a vitally important part of the recovery process.

Finding Treatment Options

As I promised, there are a variety of treatment options available for people who are bulimic. I mention them briefly here and suggest you look in the appendix, where I list several excellent resources for locating and contacting treatment facilities and clinics around the country, as well as contact information for support groups and different types of therapeutic methods.

Treatment centers. Specialty treatment centers offer bulimics and other people with eating disorders a supportive environment where they can receive one-on-one therapy sessions and nutritional guidance. Some facilities offer both inpatient (residential) and outpatient services; others specialize in one or the other. Residential housing is another option and is for helping individuals gradually integrate back into daily life once intensive treatment is complete.

Group therapy. Group therapy is a treatment method that can take place as part of an inpatient or outpatient program or in a therapist's office, or it can be an independent entity. Some groups differ in their goals and methods and in who facilitates it (a therapist, medical professional, or layperson).

Individual counseling. This type of counseling is available both as part of a facility's treatment program and in private practice and can be done alone or in conjunction with group therapy and/or family therapy. Professionals who offer individual counseling include psychiatrists (PhD), psychologists (Psy.D or PhD), licensed clinical social workers (LCSW), certified eating disorder specialists (CEDS, if they are available in your area), and licensed professional counselors (LPC; same as a marriage and family therapist in some states). Counselors typically specialize in one or more types of therapy, such as cognitive-behavioral therapy, psychoanalysis, and Jungian therapy.

12-Step programs. These groups are typically spiritually based and involve the concept of sponsors or a "buddy" system. Twelve-step groups are frequently used by bulimics as part of their long-term recovery process.

Workshops. Some treatment facilities, clinics, and programs offer periodic workshops for people who are in recovery. These workshops can be residential or nonresidential, and often focus on relapse prevention.

Complementary therapies. This category includes therapy methods that are best used *along with* one or more conventional methods. Many people find that including complementary approaches enhances their recovery process. Some of the complementary therapies include art therapy, breathing therapy, Feldenkrais Method, life coaching, meditation, reiki, spiritual guidance, tai chi, and yoga.

Hospitalization. "I don't want to go to a hospital!" After a few weeks of discussions with her mother, sixteen-year-old Melody had finally agreed to get help for bulimia, but she was adamant about not going to a hospital. In her case, hospitalization was not necessary. In fact, hospitalization is usually a last resort rather than the first for people with bulimia. It is critical, however, for individuals whose weight is dangerously low and/or who have a serious physical condition stemming from purging, such as a ruptured esophagus or gastrointestinal bleeding. Once any in-hospital stay is complete, the bulimic can enter an appropriate treatment program. Typically, plans for such a treatment program are put into motion while the patient is in the hospital and may even begin during hospitalization.

BOTTOM LINE

In this chapter I discussed the first step to recovery, which is twofold: how to identify and acknowledge bulimia; and how to help a bulimic accept the need for treatment. I set the stage for the different types of treatment available for bulimics, and now you are ready to explore them in more depth.

CHAPTER 6

STEP 2: LET TREATMENT BEGIN!

Congratulations! You're ready for step 2. Whether you're a bulimic or an individual who is helping someone dear to you, this chapter can guide you through the process of initiating and participating in treatment. By now you realize that bulimia is *not* about food, that it is a multifaceted disease, and that it requires a comprehensive, multidisciplinary approach to treatment that includes attention to both emotional and physical (medical and dietary) needs. However, unless there is an acute or pressing medical condition that requires immediate attention, the first thing you need to do—with the help of professionals—is aggressively address the emotional issues that are driving you or your loved one to binge and purge.

If you are bulimic, you may say to yourself, "I don't need help. I can beat this disease by myself." Or you may say, "Tomorrow is a new day, and I won't binge or purge," or "If I only eat this, then I won't binge," or "If I keep myself real busy then I won't want to binge and purge." Although your intentions may be good, can you honestly say that any of these attempts have worked? Although "giving in" to getting professional help may *seem* like you are relinquishing control, the truth is that if none of these efforts have been successful, then you don't have control now. The disease has control of you. To regain true control of your life, you need guidance from people who understand and work with bulimia. Just keep in mind that this is a team effort, and that the goal is your health.

Singer Katharine McPhee certainly found the relief she needed from experts, and in a big way. The twenty-two-year-old "American

Idol" runner-up announced in June 2006 that she had struggled with bulimia for years, throwing up as many as seven times a day for five years, before she sought help. Her motivation for seeking therapy was her successful audition for "American Idol," after which she became very worried that throwing up was damaging her vocal cords and would ruin her chances for a singing career. She immediately enrolled in an eating disorder facility and participated in both group and individual therapy sessions six days a week for three months. She told reporters for *People* magazine in an interview that was published on the publication's website that she believes she's healthier now because of the "intuitive eating" method she learned in therapy.

Intuitive eating is just one of the methods I discuss in this chapter, where you will learn more about various approaches to treatment through the eyes and experiences of several people with bulimia who used these methods. Through their experiences with a variety of treatment approaches, I hope to help you get a better understanding of how they work and how they can help you or a loved one to eliminate binge/purge and other compulsive, destructive behaviors and to regain self-esteem, confidence, and joy for life.

A WORLD OF TREATMENT POSSIBILITIES

In chapter 5 I briefly mentioned some of the general approaches to treatment of bulimia, but in this chapter we will look at them in detail. Treatment methods and programs for people who have bulimia are as different and variable as the people seeking them and the facilities or therapists who offer them. Generally, however, treatment may include one or more of the following:

- Cognitive behavioral therapy
- Dialectic behavioral therapy
- Interpersonal psychotherapy
- Psychodynamic psychotherapy
- Eye movement desensitization and reprocessing
- Family therapy
- Group therapy
- Twelve-step groups and self-help
- Nutritional therapy
- Medication

"I was surprised by the number of choices I had," says Bonnie, a thirty-one-year-old part-time bookkeeper and mother of a three-year-old daughter. "I had hidden my bulimia for more than ten years, but when I got pregnant with my second child, I began to worry that something might go wrong, and I would never forgive myself. Even so, I couldn't make myself go for help, so I started visiting websites and reading about other women who had taken the steps I still couldn't make myself take. But when I read about the different therapies and how they were helping other women, I was inspired and convinced that there was something that could help me. I went to my doctor, told her what I had read, and together we chose a treatment plan that allowed me to stay at home with my daughter and still get intensive therapy sessions and nutritional help. I'm happy to say that Sean was born healthy and perfect, that I'm in recovery, and that I still get wonderful help from a support group that I attend weekly."

WHERE DO I GO FROM HERE?

Crystal's biggest fear was that she would have to go to a hospital; Cliff was afraid he would lose his job if he went into full-time treatment; Abbie didn't want to be away from her children; Dawn was concerned about missing her college classes. All of them worried that they would have to give up control, even though what they had was a false sense of control and bulimia was actually controlling them.

All of these feelings are real, valid concerns that people with bulimia wrestle with when they think about getting treatment. They want to be able to continue to do the things that are meaningful and maintain structure in their lives while they get help. Fear that treatment will take away or dramatically change what is dear to them is a major reason why some people avoid seeking treatment. Chances are, you or a loved one is wrestling with these concerns and fears as well. Let's begin to erase them here and now!

Treatment Venue Options

Fortunately, not only are there a variety of therapeutic options from which you can choose, but you can also work with professionals to create your own plan that fits your needs and lifestyle. Also, patients typically find that treatment is more intense in the beginning and gradually becomes less so with time. There are four general treatment options listed in descending order of intensity.

Hospitalization, in a community hospital or medical center. As I mentioned previously, most bulimics do not need to be hospitalized. However, individuals whose weight is dangerously low (especially seen among people who are both anorexic and bulimic) and/or who require intravenous fluids, cardiac care, or other medical interventions, may need hospitalization for a short time until their medical condition is stabilized. Hospitalization in a psychiatric facility is also indicated for people who are suicidal.

If hospitalization is required, it is strongly recommended that psychiatric care also be initiated simultaneously, as this is the primary type of treatment bulimics need once they are released from the hospital. Because hospitalization and beginning psychiatric treatment can be frightening and alien to many people, everything possible should be done to minimize these feelings. Thus beginning psychiatric care in the hospital will make the transition out of the hospital easier and offers patients a sense of security and continuity.

One mistake well-intentioned people often make is that they use the possibility of hospitalization as a threat or as a treatment of last resort. "If you don't stop throwing up, you'll have to be admitted to the hospital" is perceived as a threat to many bulimics, as it was to sixteen-year-old Vivian. "I can look back now and see that my parents meant well," says Vivian, who is now nineteen and a college student.

"I was bulimic and anorexic and throwing up three to four times a day when my parents delivered their threat," she says. "I was terrified of hospitals because my little brother had died in one after a car accident when I was five years old, so their warning just made me dig in my heels even more." Eventually Vivian entered an inpatient facility for 30 days but did not need to be hospitalized.

Inpatient Eating Disorder Facility (Residential Facility). Bulimics often do not require intensive medical care, yet they need treatment and supervision on a twenty-four-hour-per-day basis. The answer to this need is an inpatient eating disorder (aka residential) facility. The main goal of treatment at a residential facility is to help individuals gain control over their bingeing and purging so they can move forward to more "normal" eating (and exercising) habits. Scores of such facilities are available in North America (see appendix). Most residential facilities have doctors and nurses readily available, although often they are on-call rather than onsite. A stay at an inpatient facility can range from a few days to several weeks, months, or longer. The length of stay depends on the clients' needs (residents are usually referred to as "clients" and not as "patients" because they do not require acute medical care) and on how they progress with the programs the facility offers.

Donna, a thirty-two-year-old hotel manager, checked out several residential treatment centers in her state before she chose one that was an hour's drive from her home.

"I was bulimic for fifteen years before I decided to get help," says Donna, "and during that time I swore I would quit on many different occasions. It never worked. I finally realized I was cheating my daughter and husband out of quality time, and I was cheating myself as well. I knew I needed twenty-four-hour help, and that I had to go to a residential facility to get it. Once I was there, I realized how naïve I had been. There was no way I could have resolved the complex emotions I had suppressed without professional help. During the process I also discovered that I was regaining control, not giving it up. And that feeling really helped me with the healing process. I was in the facility for one month, and it turned my life around."

Residential centers typically offer nutritional counseling, one or more forms of psychiatric therapy (e.g., individual, group, family), and medication monitoring, but they differ in regards to other services provided, number of clients served, type of payment plans they will accept, and length of programs offered. Some facilities, such as the Eating Disorder Center in Denver, for example, offer clients an opportunity to shop for food, plan meals, cook, and engage in other daily activities that typically are problem areas for bulimics. The chance to practice these activities in a residential facility can provide individuals with valuable skills and help them take increasing responsibility for their own health and well-being. Some residential centers offer specialized services, such as acupuncture, homeopathy, yoga, meditation, and massage; many are qualified to treat other conditions that frequently accompany bulimia and other eating disorders, such as alcoholism or drug abuse; some are biblically or spiritually based.

Because the variety and extent of services provided by various residential treatment programs vary considerably, it is important to take some time to investigate each facility you are considering. Consult with your doctor as well as your psychiatrist, psychologist, or therapist about the types of treatment and support services you or your loved one needs and the ability of each facility to offer them. If possible, talk to former clients and/or their families about their experiences with the facility, and look for any articles or news stories that may have been written about the program or its staff. (The Internet is good for this task. You can do a global search as well as search the archives of your local newspapers.)

Day (or Night) Treatment (Partial Inpatient Program). This is a plan for people who need more structure than an outpatient program (see below) can provide but who do not need twenty-four-hour supervision or care. Day treatment is frequently the transitional step for patients who have been in an inpatient program and have "graduated," but who are not ready to go home full time and begin outpatient treatment. Typically people attend the treatment program during the day and return home at night. Day programs come in various forms: some are offered for four to five hours every day, others are held for two or three full days a week; still others are held in the evening to accommodate people who need to work during the day.

Day treatment programs are popular because they are flexible and allow people to continue to maintain intimate ties with those structures in their lives that are important—family, work, college classes, church. Services offered by day programs typically include support and supervision of two meals (one meal if it is a night program), nutritional education (preferably by a licensed dietitian or nutritionist), daily individual, group, and/or family therapy sessions, skills training (e.g., meal planning, shopping for nutritious foods, healthy exercise programs), medical evaluation by a nurse at each session, and in some cases, school lessons for adolescent patients so they will not fall behind in their school work. Day treatment programs typically last one to two months.

Intensive Outpatient Therapy. This therapeutic approach is the most flexible of the structured treatment options. Participants are typically individuals who function well during the day, but who find they need some support during the evening, when it is often more difficult to cope with or control disordered behavior. Intensive outpatient programs usually hold meetings three times a week for several hours per session. Program services offered by different facilities vary in intensity and scope, but most provide a meal with therapeutic support, therapy groups, discussion on how to refine coping skills and prevent relapse, and help with developing healthy eating patterns. Some include relaxation and stress management exercises and nutritional information programs as well. Clients typically participate for three to four weeks, but may repeat a program if they feel they need additional support.

Online and Phone Support. First, let me mention that this approach is *not* the preferred way to get treatment for bulimia; live, one-on-one personal interaction between a bulimic and his or her doctor, psychotherapist, and nutritionist, along with family therapy if needed, is the most effective way. But because people with bulimia or other eating disorders live and deal with denial, guilt, and shame, some of them who would not otherwise seek treatment are turning to online and telephone help (I discuss the value of these approaches during recovery in chapter 9). If you are not willing or able to participate in live therapy, online professional support is an option. However, **these sources are NOT treatment and should be viewed as an intermediary step: you should use the information and support you receive from them to answer your questions and to help you find a formal treatment approach that fits your needs.**

Several eating disorder organizations offer phone and online support services; I provide a list of them, with contact information, in the Appendix.

Ongoing Support. This category does not include structured programs, but I include it here to let you know that help and support do not end once one has "graduated" from intensive outpatient therapy: there are sources of ongoing support that recovering bulimics can access whenever they feel the need to do so. I discuss the area of ongoing support in detail in chapter 8. You may be surprised at how much support there is!

TYPES OF THERAPY

The menu of therapeutic options for bulimics is varied, as you'll see below, although not all types of therapy may be available in a given area and/or offered by the facility you have chosen. However, it is a good idea to familiarize yourself with the options so you can make a more informed decision when it comes time for treatment.

Cognitive Behavioral Therapy

Cognitive behavioral therapy (CBT) is a psychotherapy approach in which individuals learn how to take control of their lives and their illness by recognizing their distorted, irrational thinking and learning how to replace those unhealthy thoughts with positive, more realistic ones. For bulimics, this usually means discovering new ways to think about their body, eating habits, meal planning, nutrition, and dieting, and any fears they have about food, weight, and body image, as well as new ways to behave.

Of the many types of psychotherapy available, cognitive behavioral therapy is believed by many experts to be the best approach for people who have bulimia nervosa. Studies show that it is more effective than various other therapies, and it is usually the first approach therapists use when initiating treatment for bulimics.

In a head-to-head comparison of CBT and interpersonal psychotherapy (see below), 220 patients with bulimia were randomly assigned to receive 19 sessions of either CBT or interpersonal therapy for 20 weeks and then evaluated one year later. Immediately after treatment ended, CBT was significantly better than interpersonal psychotherapy (45% recovered vs. 8% recovered, respectively), but at one-year follow-up, the percentages had drawn much closer together, to 40 percent and 27 percent, respectively. This study shows that cognitive-behavioral therapy provides more rapid improvement as compared with interpersonal psychotherapy, but that in the long-run (at one year at least), both types of therapy had similar results.

One of the features of cognitive behavioral therapy that appeals to many patients—besides the fact that it's very effective—is that it's fairly short. "I was surprised to hear that my therapy sessions would last about five months," says Francine, a twenty-five-year-old bank teller. "I was so afraid I would have to be in therapy for years, so when the therapist explained that I would have one session a week for 18 to 20 weeks, I was very happy."

Cognitive behavior therapists who work with bulimics focus on changing eating behaviors to include more flexible and healthy eating habits, and learning coping skills to prevent bingeing and purging. Therapy also includes learning how to cope with stress and negative thinking, and on those thoughts and feelings that can trigger bingeing and purging.

"I used to have an endless tape running in my head," says Tod, a twenty-two-year-old software writer and competitive runner, "and it was always telling me that I wasn't good enough, that I could always do better than I was doing, and that I didn't deserve anything better in life. I always felt like I was on the edge of a binge, twenty-four-hours a day." Tod began working with a psychotherapist during his stay at a day treatment facility, and he noticed a change in his attitude after just a few sessions. "My therapist and I worked on new ways for me to cope with stress and negative moods rather than bingeing," explains Tod. "We met only once a week, but every day in between I was using everything I learned in my sessions—how to switch off the negative talk in my head and replace it with positive thoughts and actions and thus prevent a binge." Tod stayed in a day facility for three weeks before he graduated to an intensive outpatient therapy program, but he kept seeing his psychotherapist for CBT once a week for an additional 17 weeks. By the end of the 20 weeks, Tod and his therapist had developed strategies for Tod to prevent a relapse, cope with stressful situations, and stay with healthy eating habits.

Dialectic Behavioral Therapy

Dialectic behavioral therapy (DBT) is a modified form of cognitive behavioral therapy, and it was originally designed to help individuals who self-harm are suicidal, and/or whose emotions are out of control. The motto of DBT is to create "lives worth living." The technique has been used successfully with bulimics and people who binge eat. Dialectic behavioral therapy focuses on four stages of treatment with target goals that help clients to:

- Cease their out-of-control behavior and move to being in control. Various techniques are used to help bulimics regain control of their eating patterns (see below).
- Move from being emotionally shut down to experiencing their emotions fully. Since bulimia is about emotions and not about food, this is a critical step in the therapeutic process.
- Build an ordinary life and solve ordinary problems. Examples may include learning how to solve marital problems, difficulties with one's children, or work dissatisfaction.
- Move from a feeling of being incomplete to one of completeness. This may involve changing jobs, finding a life partner, or making a spiritual connection.

Therapists help clients reach these targets through three main techniques: individual therapy (usually conducted for 60 to 90 minutes once per week), skills group sessions (two-hour sessions once per week), and telephone support. In the skills group, clients learn about mindfulness, interpersonal effectiveness, emotion regulation, and distress tolerance. The telephone support aspect of DBT appeals to many clients, because it offers them a safety net in between therapy sessions. Clients are urged to call their therapist if and when they have an uncontrollable urge to self-harm or to binge and purge so the therapist can talk them through what they are feeling and hopefully help them avoid the harmful behavior.

A group of 28 women with bulimia were part of a randomized controlled study that noted just how effective dialectic behavioral therapy can be. The participants were assigned to receive either 20 weeks of DBT or to a waiting list (they received no therapy at the time, but were promised treatment once the study was completed). The treated women attended weekly 50-minute individual psychotherapy sessions during which they learned emotional regulation skills that would help them replace their bingeing and purging. At the end of the 20 sessions, four of the fourteen treated women had stopped bingeing and purging completely, five had dramatically reduced (by 88%) their disordered eating behaviors, and five had not improved. Two of the women in the waiting group had some improvement, but twelve did not.

Interpersonal Therapy

Interpersonal therapy is an approach in which clients and therapists focus on understanding the links between interpersonal relationship problems, depression, and/or anxiety, and eating disorder episodes. This therapy does not focus on body image, food intake, or weight at all. Rather, the goals of therapy are to: (1) express emotions and feelings; (2) develop independence and a strong sense of self; (3) learn how to tolerate and cope with change and uncertainties; and (4) face any traumatic issues from the past that may be contributing to disordered eating and behaviors.

For example, therapy might focus on the problems bulimics have forming or maintaining relationships, disputes they are having with family members or friends, fears about career choices, past sexual or emotional abuse, or unresolved grief. Like CBT, interpersonal therapy is usually short-term and goal oriented. It can be done either individually or in a group setting. As I mentioned above in the CBT discussion, research shows that interpersonal therapy is almost as effective as CBT in treating bulimia over the long-term, although CBT provides faster results. Some therapists use a combination of the two therapies, which has proved effective in at least one study.

Psychodynamic Therapy

Psychodynamic therapy is a general term for an approach that helps individuals explore their subconscious and identify feelings that have been too painful to face, with the goal being to help them deal and cope with the feelings. There are several different kinds of psychodynamic therapies; some focus directly on bulimic behaviors, while other focus on the problems that underlie the eating disorder. Typically, psychodynamic therapists attempt to have clients understand and resolve conflicts that developed during their childhood. Psychodynamic therapies have not been studied as extensively as other psychotherapeutic approaches. On average, psychodynamic therapy takes longer than CBT or interpersonal therapy, and some therapists use it in conjunction with other approaches.

Eye Movement Desensitization and Reprocessing

A relatively new psychotherapy technique called eye movement desensitization and reprocessing (EMDR) is being used by some experts to help people who suffer from anxiety, panic, trauma, post-traumatic stress, and other emotional disorders. Although it has not been studied scientifically in eating disorders, some psychotherapists report that it has benefited their patients who have bulimia and other eating disorders.

The basis of EMDR is rapid eye movement, or REM. During sleep, the brain uses REM to help it process the day's emotional experiences. This process can break down when daytime trauma has been especially difficult or extreme, which means REM sleep doesn't provide sufficient relief from the stress. EMDR is the next step in REM processing. Here's how some experts believes it works.

When trauma occurs, memory of the event is stored in the brain. However, because the brain of a traumatized person appears to be unable to process the experiences normally, the memories and feelings of the event become stuck in the nervous system, where they cause distress and in turn upset normal emotional functioning.

In the late 1980s, psychologist Francine Shapiro, PhD, noted that specific eye movements reduced the severity of disturbing thoughts in some of her clients. This finding lead her to conduct scientifically based research which in turn resulted in the method she called EMDR. The technique she developed releases the negative memories and emotions that are stored in the nervous system and then helps the brain process the experience it was unable to process previously.

To accomplish this, specially trained therapists guide their patients to remember the traumatic event. As memories of the event come to the surface, the patient's eye movements are matched with the remembered events and then guided to other specific movements that then cause the memories to be released. EMDR experts say that when clients bring their memories back to the surface, they experience the feelings about them in a new way, allowing them to get a new perspective on the event and also control over the situation.

Clients continue with EMDR sessions until they have come to terms with all the traumatic memories that have been underlying their disorder. In most cases, EMDR sessions bring about positive results faster than other psychotherapy techniques, including cognitive behavioral therapy. That's because rather than concentrate on analyzing the meaning of the memories that are brought to the surface, EMDR shortens the process and helps the client release the memories and emotions. The result, say EMDR experts, is that the memory remains, but the client's negative response to it is eliminated.

EMDR can be used along with other psychotherapy techniques and help hasten the intense therapeutic part of a bulimic's recovery process. If this type of psychotherapy interests you, look for a licensed psychotherapist, psychiatrist, social worker, or counselor who has received specific EMDR training.

Family Therapy

When one person in a family has an eating disorder, especially when that person is a child or adolescent, the entire family is affected. What does this mean? For one thing, parents worry and ask themselves: Did we do something to contribute to this problem? Is it our fault? What can we do to help our child? Having a child with bulimia or another eating disorder places a great deal of stress on a family, and some parents find their coping skills are challenged to the max. If there are siblings at home, very often they have a difficult time understanding what is happening to their brother or sister. Sometimes siblings believe they're responsible for their brother or sister being sick, or they may act out and rebel against any additional attention being given to the bulimic child.

A family therapist can be a safe place for family members to turn for explanations and answers to their questions about bulimia and its impact on each individual. In family therapy sessions, the interrelationships of family members are explored to help identify and resolve any problems or conflicts family members are having. A family therapist guides family members through their emotional changes as they learn to cope with the therapeutic process the bulimic is experiencing and what it means to the rest of the family. Most therapists agree that family therapy is a necessary part of any comprehensive psychological treatment of bulimia and other eating disorders.

There are several different types of family therapies. One, called structural family therapy, focuses on members' roles in the family as well as any conflicts and other family dynamics and how they all may relate to the eating disorder. Factors such as poor communication among family members, family values that highlight the importance of weight and appearance, and an inability to deal with emotions may all contribute to or interfere with recovery from bulimia.

Valerie and her seventeen-year-old daughter, Monica, as well as Monica's eleven-year-old sister Celia began attending weekly family therapy sessions the week after Monica was admitted to an inpatient facility for bulimia. Monica had been bingeing and purging for about two years before she entered the program. Valerie says she was surprised—and heartened—by the whole family therapy process and how helpful it was.

"I thought I was going to be made to feel like Monica's illness was my fault, that because I was a single mom I had somehow neglected my child's emotional and physical well-being," says Valerie. "But I did learn that I had been unintentionally emphasizing appearance and dieting and not focusing on higher values, like what an incredibly kind and talented person Monica is. During therapy sessions I also came to realize that Celia was also tending toward an eating disorder, and I was so grateful that Celia and I were able to identify that and nip it in the bud. The sessions were tough, but invaluable for our family and for Monica."

Another form of family therapy is family-based treatment, which usually can be completed in a shorter amount of time (about 20 sessions) than structural therapy, and is especially suitable when the bulimic is a child or adolescent. This form of therapy focuses on helping the parents temporarily take charge of their child's disordered eating and helping the child regain his or her own control. Once the bulimic behavior can be managed, the parents return control over eating back to the child and assist him or her to develop normal, healthy eating habits and ways to manage stress.

Group Therapy

Group therapy is typically part of inpatient and outpatient treatment programs and is run or moderated by a professional psychologist or other qualified health professional. Some people say group therapy is a bit frightening at first, because it involves exposing themselves in front of others. When individuals relax and give group therapy a chance, however, many find that it can be very helpful.

Geoff was very apprehensive about going to group therapy during his stay in residential treatment. "I swore I wasn't going to like it," says this twenty-three-year-old graduate student. "I admit I was a bit defiant at first. But then as I listened to the others, I felt a kinship, less isolated. I thought to myself, 'hey, that sounds like me talking,' and I felt better about the whole experience. I didn't participate in the discussion the first few times I went to group, but by the third session I was talking. The group leader was very supportive, and I felt safe, never judged for what I was saying."

In group therapy, bulimics learn that they are not the only ones who have certain fears, anger, doubts, and other strong emotions. Group therapy gives them an opportunity to share their fears and questions with others, in the company of a psychologist or other professional, in a safe environment. Group therapy can help bulimics (1) learn more about the emotional conflicts that are behind their abnormal eating behaviors, (2) share their fears, problems, and coping strategies with others, (3) develop a healthy relationship with food and realize reasonable weight goals, and (4) improve their ability to communicate with others.

12-Step Groups and Self-Help Methods

Professional treatment, as outlined above, should be the first and primary approach whenever possible. No one knows how many bulimics recover without professional therapy or without significant help from his or her family, but it seems unlikely that most people can recover completely without at least some expert assistance. That being said, participation in twelve-step groups (e.g., Eating Disorders Anonymous, Overeaters Anonymous) and attempts at self-help, including other self-help groups and self-help books and manuals, can certainly be useful components of the recovery process and complement those efforts.

Sometimes individuals are ready to pursue treatment but the facility they have chosen or the psychotherapist they want to see isn't immediately available. Rather than wait, starting the treatment process by attending a 12-step group and/or following a self-help manual can fill the gap until more structured, professional treatment can begin.

This idea was tested in an eight-week study by a group of experts who examined the effectiveness of unguided self-help as a first step in the treatment of bulimia. Eighty-five women who were on a waiting list for hospital-based treatment were randomly assigned to receive either a self-help manual (one on cognitive behavior self-help or one on self-assertion skills) or to a waiting list. Slightly more than half of the patients in the self-help group reported at least a 50 percent reduction in bingeing and purging as compared with the waiting list group (31 percent). The patients in the self-help group did not show any significant changes in their levels of concern about body shape, weight, or eating or in their general emotional state, however.

In another study, 62 patients were randomly assigned to use a self-care manual along with eight sessions of cognitive behavioral therapy (an approach termed "guided self-help) or to participate in 16 sessions of weekly cognitive behavioral therapy alone. At the end of the treatment period and up to an average of 43 weeks after the end of treatment, patients in both groups had substantial improvement in their disordered eating behaviors. In fact, 71 percent of those in the CBT group had not binged or vomited during the week before follow-up, and in the guided self-help group, 70 percent had not binged and 61 percent had not vomited during the week before follow-up. This study showed that guided self-help could be as effective as CBT in people with bulimia.

Twelve-step groups and self-help approaches can arguably be used throughout the treatment process. Many people, for example, use 12-step groups and self-help methods as support mechanisms once they have graduated from more formal treatment in a facility or outpatient program. For that reason, I revisit these treatment approaches in chapter 8, where I talk about recovery tools, and discuss how they can be useful at this stage of the healing process.

Nutritional Therapy

It's necessary for bulimics to establish a trusting, comfortable relationship with a nutritionist or dietician so they can feel safe as they recover from their eating disorder. Regular counseling from a dietician or nutritionist who is familiar with bulimia is typically part of any reputable treatment program, whether it's an inpatient or outpatient plan. Inpatient, residential programs usually provide daily nutritional therapy and support, while less structured programs, including outpatient programs, may offer nutritional guidance once a week or less often.

Some of the features of bulimia and other eating disorders include unrealistic fears about food, and the loss of the ability to recognize what "normal eating" is. A nutritionist or dietician who specializes in bulimia and other eating disorders can help their clients establish a foundation for a nutritious and balanced eating plan, which is essential to recovery. "I was convinced that if I just looked at a piece of cake, I would gain 10 pounds," says Hannah. "And I know intellectually that that is a ridiculous statement, but that's what I believed. I was afraid of a piece of cake. I was afraid of a lot of different foods."

Fear of food is something bulimics need to overcome as part of the healing process. A nutritionist who is familiar with bulimia can help clients overcome these feelings. People who use food as a coping mechanism, as bulimics do, often find that changing their habits—bingeing, vomiting, exercising excessively, misusing laxatives—can be terrifying. Part of the job of a nutritionist (as well as a psychotherapist) is to help bulimics establish a normal relationship with food and eating and to let go of the power they allow food to have over them. This work often includes helping clients overcome their fears about eating one or more foods they believe are especially "dangerous," like the piece of cake Hannah was convinced would make her gain ten pounds.

"My nutritionist worked very hard to convince me that eating a single piece of cake would not thrust ten pounds of ugly fat on my hips," says Hannah. "For weeks, I felt sheer panic at the thought of putting a single morsel of cake into my mouth. She brought out the scientific evidence; she talked about metabolism and how I would need to consume 3,500 calories more than I burned in order to gain even one pound." Many nutritionists ask their clients to keep a food diary, which allows bulimics and nutritionists to evaluate current eating habits and to help bulimics improve their food choices.

A nutritionist who is an expert on eating disorders can also help bulimics reconnect with the social aspect of eating, such as dining in restaurants, sharing meals with family and friends, and attending social occasions at which food is served. All of these activities can be very painful for people with bulimia, so one goal of nutritional therapy is to help them lose the fear and rigidity they have when they are in such situations.

Medications

Bulimia isn't like a headache: you can't take a pill to make it go away. However, a physician or psychiatrist can prescribe medications—primarily antidepressants—to assist with the recovery process. Notice that I say, "assist," as medications cannot cure bulimia or other eating disorders, but they can be used to alleviate the depression, anxiety, or related symptoms that often accompany them and thus facilitate the recovery process. For people with bulimia or binge eating disorder, several medications can be helpful. Here's a brief summary of the drugs used in the treatment of bulimia. Drugs are most effective when they are used in conjunction with psychotherapy and nutrition counseling. If your doctor prescribes any of these medications, please be sure he or she (and/or your pharmacist) explains the side effects, cautions, and any possible drug and/or herb interactions to you. I also recommend you consult the latest edition of the *Physician's Desk Reference* (available in most libraries in the reference section) for information about any medications you take.

Fluoxetine (Prozac). A short-term clinical trial has shown this selective serotonin reuptake inhibitor (SSRI) to be effective in reducing the symptoms of bulimia and helping patients avoid a relapse by the end of one year.

Lithium. This is an antipsychotic drug that is useful in bulimia as well as bipolar disorder, a condition that occurs in some people with eating disorders.

Desipramine (Norpramin). Desipramine is a tricyclic antidepressant used to treat bulimia, depression, and panic disorder.

Naltrexone (Revia). This drug was approved by the FDA for treatment of alcoholism but not for treatment of bulimia, although some physicians prescribe it for this off-label use because it's been shown to be effective. It may also be helpful in treating bulimics who engage in self-harm.

Imipramine (Tofranil). This tricyclic antidepressant is approved for depression but is also given for bulimia and panic disorder.

Ondansetron (Zofran). This drug is approved for reducing the nausea and vomiting that often accompanies cancer chemotherapy. Ondansetron works by reducing the activity of the vagus nerve, the nerve that transmits signals between the brain and the stomach and lets people know when they've had enough to eat. Some researchers suggest that at least in some bulimics, bingeing and vomiting are caused by over stimulation of the vagus nerve, and thus ondansetron, which suppresses that activity also decreases the urge to binge and purge.

BOTTOM LINE

In this chapter you learned about the first line of defense when it comes to treatment, and that defense involves psychotherapy— inpatient or outpatient—in one or more forms, along with medical attention if needed. Once you or your loved one has made a firm commitment to such therapy and is well on the road to recovery, it's time to restore the smile that so many bulimics have had to hide. This is an exciting part of the process for me, and I'm anxious to tell you about it.

CHAPTER 7

STEP 3: LEARNING TO SMILE AGAIN

Tears. Exclamations of joy. And more tears. This is a typical response from my patients when they get their first look at the finished product: the restoration work on their teeth and gums that has brought back their smile. I'm always thrilled to be able to erase much or all of the devastating damage that purging has done to the teeth, gums, and mouth of people with bulimia. But the real power of the restoration work is much more than cosmetic: restoring a bulimic's smile and oral health has a tremendous positive impact on a patient's emotional well-being: their self-esteem, confidence, hope for the future, feelings of worth, and the will and courage to continue treatment.

In this chapter I take you on a journey: from the moment I and my staff first make contact with a bulimic patient, through the interview process, and how we establish the relationship with the patient in preparation for the restorative dental work. I then explain the type of restorative work I and other dentists can offer patients who have lived with bulimia or purging disorder. I also invite you to visit several websites where you can see the before-and-after photographs of the smiles of people with bulimia and also hear comments from patients and their experiences with the restoration process: see my own website, *www.acld.com* or *www.bulimiaisadentaldisease.org* for stories on eating disorders and real life before and after photographs.

Learning to Smile Again: The Journey Begins

When I first became actively involved in helping my bulimic patients acknowledge their eating disorder and agree to seek professional treatment, I usually uncovered the disorder during the initial dental examination. In the last few years, however, our reputation for dealing with these patients in a caring and professional manner has grown, until today it is more common to have patients tell my office staff over the phone or during the initial interview (before I conduct the dental examination) that they have an eating disorder, and that the reason for their visit is to correct the problems it has caused.

Below I explain my general approach to working with patients who are bulimic or who have purging disorder.

The Initial Interview

An element critical to our success, I believe, is the initial interview. The purpose of the first meeting is to allow patients to explain their hopes, desires, and needs concerning their dental health before we get into a detailed discussion of the type of work they will need to achieve those goals. Our treatment coordinator conducts the interview, which is done in a non-threatening, non-clinical setting; in fact, patients say they feel like they're in our living room. That's because there's no imposing front desk and filing cabinets; just comfortable, family room furniture and lit aromatherapy candles. We make every effort to minimize any anxiety or apprehension associated not only with making a dental visit, which is stressful enough for many people, but also the feelings around trying to hide or finally admit one has an eating disorder.

During that initial interview, our treatment coordinator allows patients all the time they need to feel safe, comfortable, and relaxed. Our goal is to establish open, honest communication and a trust-bond relationship. Such a relationship makes it much more likely that a bulimic patient will admit her eating disorder to us, and it facilitates the treatment process as well. Once it becomes clear that there is a rapport between the patient and the coordinator, we can all move forward and address the reason the patient came to us in the first place. This is when I join the meeting and conduct the dental examination.

If a patient has already admitted her bulimia to us, it is easy to take the next steps. We can discuss the type of professional help she needs and/or is getting and then make arrangements for her dental work to begin. If a bulimic patient has not admitted she has a problem, our course is more challenging. Once I conduct my examination, I dismiss the treatment coordinator, sit the patient up, pull my chair around so I can be face to face with the patient, and get honest.

"I've found some teeth that I have concerns about, and I need some more information. Is it OK if I ask you a few questions?" No one has ever answered no to that question. "The condition of your teeth is similar to the condition of others who have an eating disorder. Do you now or have you ever had an eating disorder?" The odds are in my favor: my experience is that more than 50 percent of the time patients admit they are or were bulimic.

If the patient admits to the bulimia, she has placed a great deal of trust in me, and I cannot break that trust by being judgmental in any way. I also cannot assume she is ready to seek outside professional help for the bulimia. Thus my mission at this point is to be empathic and help the patient believe she can trust me and that I am concerned about her overall health.

Once a patient has admitted to the eating disorder, I can begin to ask a series of questions: How long has she been dealing with her eating disorder? Does she have any other symptoms or issues? Has she sought help or guidance from other professionals? Does she need a referral to a physician or counselor? Is this the first time she has been bulimic, is she a relapsed patient, or a serial bulimic?

Mapping the Road to Recovery

We can then begin to map out our strategy for restoring her oral health. The road map differs for each patient, depending on if she has started treatment for the bulimia, where she is in the treatment process, and the extent of the dental damage, but it is important that we begin, to relieve both her physical and emotional turmoil. If the patient is actively in treatment, I like to consult and coordinate with the other professionals involved in her care, either in writing or by telephone. I believe it is important to keep her physician and therapist informed regarding her dental health and the positive self-esteem and overall benefits it provides. In addition, the feedback and information

I get from them can help me with my restoration work. Medication, usually antidepressants for bulimia, can influence saliva production and flow, and thus negatively impact dental health. It also helps if I have an idea of the progress of behavioral therapy, so I can better plan the stages of dental treatment.

If the patient first comes to me when she is further along in therapy and is currently in an outpatient-counseling environment, the level of trust is greater than it would be before or at the beginning of eating disorder treatment. Although trust and communication are still key, a great deal of tension and anxiety have been removed from the picture. Patients who have graduated to group therapy or one-on-one outpatient counseling are typically well on their way to resolving their major issues, and dental restoration is perhaps just one stop on their road to recovery.

Communication is Key

The key to success with any bulimic patient, regardless of where she is in her acceptance of or treatment for the disease, is communication. I strive to be clear about everything I say and to portray empathy and care at every opportunity. I watch body language and look for trust in her eyes before I move on to the next question or comment. I listen for her acceptance or dismissal of what I am saying. This emphasis on communication extends to the actual dental treatment process as well. If there are times when a patient, my assistant or I feel the patient needs a break or is in distress, I stop treatment, put down my equipment, take off my protective mask and goggles and we talk until she's calm. We may end treatment then or continue—it all depends on how everyone feels. I won't proceed unless the patient is reassured and calm.

The Power of a Smile

I can't emphasize enough the power of a healthy smile. I'm not saying this just because I'm a dentist, but because it's true. A positive self-image and self-esteem are critical for recovery from bulimia, and a restored, healthy smile is evidence of those feelings. Does having a new smile help the recovery process? Absolutely. So many patients tell me that their dental restoration work has been a life-changing event for them.

The Patient In Denial

Sometimes patients will not admit they have bulimia or purging disorder, even after I have asked them direct questions about eating disorders and talk about how their teeth show evidence of such a disease. Some of these patients are in denial to themselves; others acknowledge to themselves that they are bulimic but they are still trying to hide the disease. Those in the former category can benefit from positive reinforcement and knowing that my door is always open to discuss how they feel. Patients in the latter category are often shocked when they discover that I can detect the disease they've hidden so well from family and friends. Their body language says it all: some blush, others look away, stammer, dart their eyes, draw into themselves—they've been "caught" with their hands in the proverbial cookie jar.

For most, this is the first time they've learned how much damage they are really doing to their teeth and gums. This situation can stir up many emotions that are difficult for the patients to handle, so I must proceed with kid gloves. They feel lost, vulnerable; their defenses are down. Many need to process the fact that I've uncovered their "secret" and so continue to deny their condition, at least for the time being. Admitting it to me usually comes during the next visit, or the one after that, once we have established a trust-bond relationship.

For patients in both categories, I design a treatment plan that addresses their dental needs and that also allows me an opportunity to foster a feeling of trust and relaxation on the part of the patient. I keep a close watch on these patients and bring them into the office more frequently so I can maintain their teeth, continue to build a rapport, and see how close they are to acknowledging the disease.

There is yet one more category—the critically impaired bulimic patients whose bingeing and purging are completely out of control. These patients typically have a severe, undiagnosed medical condition that requires medical attention. Such cases are rare, but when I do encounter them, I refer them to Dr. Gregory L. Jantz, PhD, a certified eating disorder specialist and founder of The Center for Counseling and Health Resources, known affectionately as A Place of Hope by many of its clients.

The Real Deal

Basically, as I discussed in chapter 4, patients must be accountable and personally responsible for their own actions. My staff and I do everything possible to help patients acknowledge the eating disorder and move along the path of recovery. For many patients, this recovery becomes a reality, and I am thrilled with their success. If, however, patients are not willing to be accountable for the damage the disease has created in their mouth and they continue to deny that impact yet request dental care, I have an ethical and moral responsibility to treat their dental condition but I cannot help them if they are not willing to be accountable.

HOW TO RESTORE A HEALTHY SMILE

Rebuilding a healthy smile is a blessing: I'm unhappy that patients have suffered and have reached a point where they need restoration; and I'm thrilled to help them get their smile back—often a smile that is even brighter than the one they had previously, because it was so hard-won!

Such restoration takes time and effort, more or less of each depending on the patient's condition. In the following sections I discuss the various techniques I and other cosmetic and restoration dentists can use to help restore a healthy mouth and smile. No two treatment plans are alike. Based on the information I gather during the initial interview and examination and in ongoing discussions, the patient and I work together to develop and implement our strategy. The techniques discussed here are among those I can bring into play to achieve the patient's goals. Exactly which ones I use depends on the extent of the damage, where the patient is in her recovery, and how that recovery process is progressing. (For a look at some of these techniques, visit *http://www.acld.com/dental-services.php*).

Crowns

Crowns, also known as caps, are coverings that are custom made to fit over teeth to protect the remaining tooth structure. They are typically used for teeth that are beyond repair and/or because they are chipped, fractured, discolored, extensively damaged by decay, too weak to support an existing filling, or overly sensitive. Teeth that have undergone root canal usually need to be protected by a crown.

Crowns are made of natural-looking porcelain and with proper care; they can last for many years without the need for replacement. Some crowns have a metal core, which improves stability, but in the crowns I use the metal cannot be seen through the porcelain. Getting fitted for a crown takes at least two visits. During the first visit, I prepare the tooth for the crown, make a mold of the tooth, and then place a temporary crown over the prepared tooth. All of this work is done while the affected area is numb, so there is no pain. Patients who experience any discomfort as the anesthetic wears off can take a mild analgesic if there is no medical reason why they cannot. And no one leaves the office without a tooth! The temporary (acrylic) crown I cement on (using a type of cement that is designed to allow easy removal of the temporary crown) protects the tooth and gum tissues until the permanent tooth is ready.

At the next visit, I remove the temporary crown, fit the prepared crown, and check the patient's bite. If we have a perfect fit, I cement the crown to the tooth, and the procedure is complete. Sometimes patients experience some mild sensitivity to cold for a few weeks, but this subsides.

Inlays and Onlays

Inlays and onlays are used to repair rear teeth that have a mild to moderate amount of decay, or to restore cracked or fractured teeth that do not require a crown. They also can be used to replace damaged or old metal fillings. Some bulimics experience problems with their fillings because of their purging activity, and so inlays may be a solution.

Here's the difference between the two approaches. Inlays are designed to treat decay within the cusps, which are the top projections of a tooth. Onlays are used to treat decay that extends to one or more of the cusps. Most inlays and onlays are made from porcelain or composite resin, although gold may be used as well. Like crowns, two visits are required to complete the process. During the first visit, I make an impression of the affected tooth and place a temporary inlay over the tooth. When patients return for the second visit, the temporary inlay is removed and the permanent one is placed. Unlike crowns, which cover a tooth, inlays and onlays are bonded to the tooth's surface. Therefore, they are only helpful for people who have a sufficient amount of enamel on their teeth. Inlays and onlays add to the integrity of the tooth while also preventing damage from bacteria.

For patients who are candidates for inlays or onlays, their use can help patients avoid the need for more extensive and expensive treatment, such as crowns, bridges, or implants. Inlays and onlays help strengthen teeth by up to 75 percent and they can last up to 30 years.

Veneers

When patients talk about improving their smile, most mention veneers (also known as porcelain veneers). Veneers are a very popular treatment approach for chipped, discolored, or crooked teeth, as well as correction of the gap-toothed look. Besides being strong, they offer patients a natural look.

Depending on the amount of erosion to the teeth, veneers may or may not be a solution for bulimics. That's because preparation for veneers requires removing an approximately one-half millimeter layer of enamel from the front of the tooth to be veneered. Patients with insufficient enamel may need to consider a crown. If there is sufficient enamel, however, I then take a mold of the tooth, and from the mold the porcelain veneer is custom made to fit the tooth. During the next visit I place the wafer-thin veneer in place with adhesive and match the veneer for color with the surrounding teeth. Once the patient and I are pleased with the look, I harden the adhesive using a special light, and the procedure is complete.

One reason for the popularity of veneers is that they have properties that very closely resemble those of real enamel: that is, they are translucent, so when light strikes the veneer, light penetrates the tooth, like it does with tooth enamel, and reflects off the dentin, which gives teeth their shine.

Bonding

For some bulimic patients who have cracked, chipped, or discolored teeth, or teeth that are misaligned, a technique called bonding (also known as composite or tooth bonding) is an option. Bonding typically can be done during a single visit. The procedure is simple: I roughen the target tooth so the composite resin (bonding material) can adhere properly to the tooth. After I apply the resin, I shape and smooth it until the desired look is achieved, then I harden the resin with a special light. Then finally I buff and polish the bonded tooth, and the patient is ready to go.

For patients who do not have extensive tooth damage, bonding is an option that is less costly and less extensive when compared with veneers, bridges, and crowns. Because the composite resin used in bonding expands and contracts with the natural tooth, it tends to be very long lasting.

Implants

Dental implants are artificial tooth roots that are placed into the jawbone to hold a replacement tooth or bridge. Implants feel very natural and they offer patients a very secure, comfortable alternative to a conventional bridge or dentures. There are two types of implants:

- endosteal, the most common type, involves surgically inserting screws or blades into the jawbone. Each implant supports one or more prosthetic teeth.
- Subperiosteal, in which the implant is placed on top of the jaw with metal posts that protrude through the gum to hold the artificial tooth. This type of implant is often used for patients who have too little bone to support an inserted implant or patients who are not able to wear conventional dentures.

Gum Laser Treatment

Gone are the days when the treatment for periodontal (gum) disease was to scrape and scale above and below the gum line of the affected tooth. We now know that the main cause of gum disease is the biofilm that develops under the gum next to the tooth. During the initial stages of gum disease, patients typically don't experience any symptoms, even though a significant infection may have developed. Current treatment is to vaporize the infection with a laser. Once the infected tissue is gone, healthy gum tissue can grow back.

Dentures

For patients whose dental decay and other damage have resulted in their losing most or all of their teeth, dentures can give them back their teeth and smile. The need for dentures can be a hard pill to swallow for many patients, especially because most people associate dentures with "old" people. Olivia, a thirty-eight-year-old apartment manager who has been in recovery for two years, remembers how she felt when she learned she needed a denture.

"I was devastated and demoralized," she said. "I had finally admitted I needed help for my bulimia, which I had been living with for eighteen years, and I knew it would be a struggle to beat it, but I was ready to fight. When my dentist explained that I would need an upper denture, I wanted to run away and never come back. But he was great; he was very understanding and gentle, and encouraged me throughout my inpatient and outpatient therapy. Once I got the denture, it took some adjustment, but it looked great, and that gave me the confidence I needed to keep on with therapy."

Dentures are the treatment of last resort; I try to preserve as many natural teeth as possible, because saving a few teeth, even just the roots, is better than removing them all. Natural teeth help retain bone in the jaw and also can support bridges or removable partial dentures. If it is not possible to save any of the teeth, a complete or implant-supported denture is the answer.

There are four types of dentures: partial, complete, conventional, and immediate. Partial dentures act as bridges because they bridge the gap between one or more missing teeth. Complete dentures cover the entire upper or lower jaw, or both. A type of complete denture is an overdenture, which fits over a few remaining teeth. Overdentures are usually used in the lower jaw. This approach usually requires that I do root canals on the remaining teeth that will be covered. Overdentures can also be fit over implants rather than natural teeth.

A conventional full denture is placed in the patient's mouth after all the teeth have been removed and the tissues have healed, which typically takes several months. This means the patient will be without teeth for several months, which explains why this is not a popular approach. One benefit of this type of denture is that the gums and bones, which shrink after teeth are removed, are allowed time to heal and reform.

Immediate dentures are the other option. Immediate complete dentures are placed the same day any remaining natural teeth are removed. The natural healing process still occurs, but because these patients are wearing dentures, they need to have several adjustments (refitting and/or relining of the denture) over the healing period to allow for the changes in the shape of the jaw and mouth.

BOTTOM LINE

Mother Teresa said, "Peace begins with a smile," and "Every time you smile at someone, it is an action of love, a gift to that person, a beautiful thing." My colleagues and I are grateful we can help bring those gifts back to the world. Once people who have lived with bulimia or purging disorder become accountable and accept personal responsibility for their lives, the road to recovery opens wide, just like the smiles that go with the journey.

CHAPTER 8

STEP 4: A WORK IN PROGRESS

"I used to laugh at people who said they were taking life one day at a time, but now I'm doing exactly that," says Abigail, a thirty-one-year-old secretary who completed an inpatient program for bulimia in spring of 2006. "I was bulimic for half my life, and now I'm learning how to live life, literally from scratch."

Recovering from bulimia is a day-by-day process for both the individuals in recovery and anyone in their immediate circle, including life partners, parents, siblings, and friends. The recovery process is a time for making lifestyle adjustments, learning new habits, understanding feelings and emotions that may have been suppressed for many years, rebuilding relationships, and "making up for lost time."

One thing recovering bulimics have told me over the years is that **recovery is a work in progress**. "I've been in recovery for five years, and there's still a tiny part of me that wants to binge and purge," says Carmela, a thirty-one-year-old insurance auditor. "Some days the urge becomes overwhelming for a while, but I push it back, use the coping skills I learned in therapy, and it subsides. But it's still there, lurking in the background."

In this chapter, we explore what life is like for people with bulimia as they learn to recover their lost lives, as seen through the eyes of several people who are in recovery, but one individual in particular, who shares her very poignant story of her sixteen-year struggle with bulimia and now her road to recovery. We also discuss how the partners, family, and friends of recovering bulimics can learn to communicate with and relate to their loved one as she or he goes through recovery and some of the challenges and rewards they can expect during the process.

REBUILDING A LIFE

"To rebuild my life, it all came down to me answering a few key questions," says Darla, twenty-three, who battled with bulimia and anorexia for more than 6 years before she entered an outpatient program. "My therapist asked me one day, 'what are you truly passionate about? What would you do if there were no barriers in your way?' And I knew the answer: I wanted to work with dogs. I've always loved dogs, but my parents didn't want them in the house. As a kid I had to satisfy myself with visiting and playing with my friends' dogs. When I was in college I couldn't have a dog in the dorm. Now I'm in my own apartment, but dogs aren't allowed.

"So I did the next best thing," says Darla. "I signed up as a volunteer at the area animal shelter, and on weekends I walk the dogs. I absolutely love it! I look forward to it all week. In fact, I've started going on Wednesday nights too. It's really helping with my recovery. I don't think about bingeing or purging when I'm with the dogs. I'm definitely less depressed. Now I'm thinking about learning how to become a dog trainer. I have a degree in business and I'm working in computers, but it's not what I want to do. Maybe I'll open a doggie daycare center. For the first time, I'm excited about something; I'm looking forward to being healthy and to living again. And that's what recovery is all about."

One of the many people who knows what recovery from bulimia is all about, and who is anxious to share her story with others, is Aimee, a thirty-four-year-old manager at a staffing agency in California. Aimee is on a mission: to help others who are living with or who are on the road to recovery from bulimia. It's a mission she is passionate about, and it shows in her dedication to the support groups she started and moderates, and the people whom she meets with week after week and talks with over the phone.

Aimee struggled with bulimia for sixteen years before she put her feet solidly on the road to recovery. If you were to meet Aimee for the first time and knew nothing about her, you would see a beautiful, vivacious, outgoing, ambitious young woman who gives off an air of confidence and kindness. It would be hard to imagine associating words like low self-esteem, despair, and hopelessness with the person beaming back at you. Yet these and other negative emotions and feelings plagued her for about half her life.

What follows is a story of that life. Aimee agreed, in fact was delighted, to share it because she wants other bulimics and their loved ones to better understand some of the thoughts, emotions, triumphs, and surmountable challenges they may experience once they decide to take back control of their lives. Aimee's story is deeply personal, yet it is also in many ways like the story of so many others who suffer with bulimia. Some of the things she says may shock or disturb you, but they are honest, from-the-heart feelings and emotions, pulled from the place she had suppressed them for so many years. Aimee's story holds many lessons, truths, guidelines, and other useful information that bulimics and their loved ones can ponder and use during their recovery. Mostly her words are full of hope, and it indeed is her hope, and mine, that her words will help those who suffer with or love someone who has bulimia.

AIMEE'S STORY

Aimee's Dream

"At one time I often dreamed of the day when I would write a moving account of my victorious, successful recovery from bulimia. It would be a story about my tragic struggle, isolation, shame, and disgust and end with a fairy tale ending of success, health, and inspiration to others. I hoped my story would make a connection with other bulimics who still struggled with the disease and give them hope, the hope I could not find but wanted so desperately all those years in the 1990s I spent secretly searching through book stores for some words—words in books that would somehow explain my disgusting behavior, my lack of control around food. I found far too few of those stories. All the books seemed to be about anorexia; bulimia was an "also ran," the supporting actor if mentioned at all. This lack of information only served to convince me that I had to struggle alone because clearly no one was writing about it, and so no one else did what I did. Therefore, I deserved to be embarrassed about it.

Of course, I eventually learned that I was wrong about at least one thing: I was not alone. In fact, there were millions of people who did what I did. And what I did was binge and purge two, three, four, or more times a day. I also learned that the fairy tale ending was just that, a fairy tale. Not that my recovery isn't a success story; it truly is, as are the stories of many other recovering bulimics I have met over the years. It's just that the success in the story looks different than I thought it would. Different, but still oh so sweet.

For one thing, I thought recovering from bulimia would be like getting over an illness: you get a diagnosis, you get treatment, and then when treatment is over, you're cured; you've 'beat' it. But bulimia isn't like having bronchitis or the flu. Instead, it's about how to not give up living life while you're in recovery.

Nor is recovery from bulimia like recovery from drug or alcohol addiction. I know drug addicts and alcoholics who have recovered. To stay in recovery, they don't use drugs or drink. But with bulimics, the drug of choice is food, and we can't give up food, so we must learn to live with it, not by it.

The Superhuman Virus

Of course, bulimia isn't about food at all; it's about feelings and emotions, and these are the things we ultimately must learn to live and deal with. One thing I learned early in recovery is that there are certain characteristics common to most bulimics, and so like most bulimics, I am infected with the Superhuman Virus (SV): the need to be good at everything I do, and to be liked and affirmed for everything I do. My standards are exceptionally high; I am competitive and super motivated to always succeed. I want others to see me as a mover and shaker, a leader and role model, all characteristics of some of the most successful people in history. It's hard to believe that such an individual could spend hours every day secretly bingeing on food and then throwing up. It was all a coping mechanism and I was very good at it, so people rarely saw me buckle under pressure. No, I kept a smile on my face and always insisted everything was under control, which was why my family and friends never knew I was bulimic until I hit bottom.

Another facet of the SV is having difficulty asking for help. I have always admired people who are independent, self-sufficient, and who are validated for these characteristics. I myself am innovative, creative, and proactive, and I've been affirmed for these traits. But when I got into trouble and couldn't fix it by myself, I perceived this inability to be a weakness, and that I was no longer responsible, controlled, honest, feminine—you name it, and I had failed. I believed I had to be liked, valued and admired by others, or else I was worthless.

Where did these feelings come from? How did they start?

The Beginning of Bulimia

I learned to throw up by accident. I was sixteen and a competitive swimmer, and had finished a "carbo-load" meal before a big race at a swim invitational. I didn't want to be weighted down, so I just bent over and threw up. I didn't even need to put my fingers down my throat. It was all so easy. Too easy.

At around the same time, I became acutely aware that society seemed to prefer thin, beautiful women. Such women were not only more popular; they also were successful, smart, and respected. I wanted to be all those things: I wanted to go to college with high academic marks, to be popular with my teachers and peers. I also had big plans to follow in the footsteps of my model parents, who had a successful marriage. My mother was a thoughtful, supportive, perfect housewife and mother; my father, hard-working, ambitious, successful, yet morally ethical. Both of them loved and supported me in everything I did. I had all the ingredients to be nothing less than perfect.

I was terribly afraid of many things, but mostly I was afraid of disappointing my parents and of not being liked. However, because I was very perceptive, I learned how to control people's reaction to me—or so I thought. I believed that if I could make people like me—if I were attractive, supportive, fun to be around, and never depressed or needy, I could guarantee that people would approve of me. As long as people liked and approved of me, I was happy. Unfortunately, sometimes my strategy backfired, and I wasn't prepared for the disappointment. I didn't have control of the situation, and it was very painful for me. I concluded that it was my fault whenever I didn't get someone's approval and admiration; obviously there was something wrong with me. That's when I began to learn that food was comforting; it was dependable, it didn't judge me, and it took away the pain.

Yet I also faced a dilemma: to be accepted, I had to be physically beautiful, but if I ate compulsively I would jeopardize that advantage. The vicious cycle of bingeing and purging began: the anxiety, which I numbed with food, which lead to more anxiety and purging. I fell into the pattern easily. In my mind, since I was able to control nearly everything else in my life, I believed I would be able to control the bulimia as well. I just thought I liked food too much and that I had no will power. As soon as I just pulled it together, I told myself, I would be in control. All I needed was more will power.

Instead, I grew increasingly ashamed of and disgusted by my behavior. I was demoralized; I was highly self-critical and self-defeating. As the years passed, I went from being a healthy, vibrant teenager and turned into a lonely, frightened, ashamed, self-defeated young woman. But the outside world didn't see that side of me; they saw the public Aimee: strong, risk-taking, thoughtful, courageous, beautiful, athletic, funny, empathetic, and motivated. I had become an expert at projecting this image and at hiding my behaviors.

The other Aimee felt like a fraud, and more and more I began to believe that I was really the less capable, less attractive, darker of the two. If someone gave me a compliment, I wanted to scream "if you only knew the real me, you would be disgusted, you would hate me." These feelings continued throughout my four years of college and followed me into my professional life after graduation.

Coming Out

The pressure of living two lives and hating myself more and more every day had become too overwhelming to bear, so about one year after graduating from college, and while I was living at home with my parents, I decided to take the plunge and tell them about my terrible secret. I believed they suspected at that point but never addressed it, and I was absolutely sure they would all be disappointed in me and disgusted by my behavior.

I was wrong. In fact, they were loving and supportive. I entered a day patient treatment program in Boulder, Colorado, which I attended at night from 5 to 9 PM, and also went to some Overeaters Anonymous meetings as well. I remember leaving the outpatient sessions and bingeing and purging on the way home. My father, who loves me dearly and wanted so desperately for me to get well, used to yell, 'You're going to kill yourself,' and his well-intended words had the unintentional effect of making me feel even more like a failure, which fueled my bingeing and purging episodes. My father, like so many family and other loved ones of people who have bulimia, just didn't understand why I couldn't "just stop it," and that the bulimia was not about food.

I then entered an inpatient program, which I insisted on paying for myself as part of my being accountable and personally responsible. After two months, however, I ran out of money, and I had to leave treatment. Together, the two programs didn't help me to understand that the bingeing and purging was about emotions; they really just focused on trying to manage food. I emerged from that round of treatment still bulimic. However, I was so embarrassed that the programs hadn't worked that I lied to my family and told them that I was fine, that the bulimia was behind me, that I was all better. They thought I was cured; I knew it was a lie.

After the First Round of Treatment

Having to lie to my parents filled me with more shame and self-disgust. Although I learned some things from the outpatient program, the bulimia was as strong as ever. I continued to work in sales and was employed by several companies and doing pretty well, which served to fuel my eating disorder because I put a lot of stress on myself to perform. I also became an expert at hiding my bulimia. My job required that I drive a great deal, visiting clients around the county. I made it a habit of bringing bagels to my customers, but I always bought two bakers' dozens and ate half of one dozen on the way to the appointment and then the other half on the way back. I would binge in my car, purge, clean up, and go to my next appointment. I knew the location of every bathroom in the county and places where I could binge in private. Because I had an expense account for food, I felt guilty because I wasn't practicing good work ethics by doing this during work time and cheating on my expenses. This filled me with even more guilt and shame, which made me binge more. But I didn't stop.

Working in sales gave me an opportunity to meet a lot of people, and one man I met at a company I worked for turned out to be quite influential in my life. He was kind, gentle, and handsome, and

I found myself confiding in him about my bulimia. In fact, I told him details that I had never revealed to anyone, and yet he accepted me unconditionally. I remember crying and crying, wondering why he didn't run away from me. I remember asking him, "Do you know what I did today? I binged on 5,000 calories; I ate 16 chocolate bars, and a dozen bagels and half a pizza and then I threw it all up in a bathroom at the beach where the vagrants sleep. Why aren't you repulsed by me?"

And he said, "Everyone has something they have to deal with." His words made me realize for the first time that bulimia was just something I had and would have to deal with. Here was a man who believed in me and really loved me. Even though I wasn't really attracted to him, I had so little faith in myself that I thought no one else would ever love me like this man does. We got married a year later.

My bulimia actually got worse while I was with him; I went from throwing up about three times a day to five because I realized that even though I liked him a great deal, I had married him for the wrong reasons. He also had company insurance that would pay for more than half of an inpatient eating disorder treatment program. I thought, this is it: I'll get my life back. I wanted to know what it was like to be normal. I prepared to enter treatment for a second time, about four years after my first round of treatment programs.

Treatment Number 2

I entered the inpatient program and found that it indeed focused on the fact that bulimia was not about food and that I needed to dive into all the things that could have caused it. The therapists kept saying, "Let's go back to your childhood when you were raped," or "Let's look into your childhood when you were molested by an uncle." However, these things were not true in my case. In fact, I had had a wonderful childhood and loving parents, so to me, the absence of such horrible events just verified that I was weak and that I had no will power with food. The staff kept reminding me that will power had nothing to do with it, and that for me, bingeing and purging were my way of dealing with anxiety and putting pressure on myself to be perfect. Food was comforting.

It took me a long time to believe I was eating to suppress issues like other people were. I used to say horrible things like, I wish I had been raped and then I'd have a reason for my bulimia. Or I said I wished I was dealing with a drug addiction so I could just stop doing it. But you can't just stop eating.

The treatment program lasted for one month, and I didn't throw up the entire time. Of course, the staff made it virtually impossible to do so, because you are watched constantly. For example, you go to the bathroom with a nurse and sing happy birthday because when you're singing you can't throw up. Because I wasn't able to suppress my feelings with food as I had done for so long, I started experiencing my emotions for the first time in many years. I realized I ate over the smallest anxiety. Being late was huge anxiety for me, because I believed that people who are perfect and professional don't run late. If I went to an appointment and was late, I would binge afterwards. I was bingeing and purging 5 times a day, and that was really challenging, but I had become an expert at it. I thought about the few occasions when I almost got caught and how for the few days after a close-call I would be so afraid and paranoid about being discovered that I would binge and purge even more.

I completed the program and began to face my feelings and realized I didn't love my husband. I needed to get well for me and get my life back. I think I married him because he loved me like I couldn't love myself. We attended couples therapy and tried to work through our situation, but eventually we got a divorce. As for post-treatment, I was following a meal plan, using many of the stress-release techniques—breathing, journaling, relaxation exercises, and many others—to help me through each day. But somehow it wasn't enough, and with a painful divorce hanging over me, I spiraled down once again.

Third Time is the Charm

On this downward spiral, I turned to something new: drugs. I found that cocaine, and then speed, were a source of temporary escape from the hate and disappointment I had in myself. The drugs kept me from bingeing for days, but when I came down, I ate for hours. I didn't know how much more I could take when out of the blue; an angel named Brenda called me. She was the director of specialty programs for Kaiser Permanente, and she called to tell me about a new, 13-week program that was covered 100 percent by insurance. My name came up because her files showed that I had been in and out of Kaiser's eating disorder therapy facilities for many years and showed no signs of progress. Was I interested?

I had to make a life-changing decision, and so I quit my job and told my mom (I still could not face my father) that I was going to enter treatment for four months, not only for bulimia but now also for amphetamine abuse. In order to keep my apartment, I used my savings to cover the rent for four months and entered intensive treatment from 7:30 AM to 4:30 PM daily.

The cliché is true: the third time is the charm. For the first time, new thought processes started to sink in. Now, as I look back, I can compare it to learning a new language: you can read it in class, speak it with fellow students, but when you go back to the "real" world, everyone is speaking English, so it's easy to drift away from what you've learned. If, however, you immerse yourself in the culture of another country while you are living your life, you can truly learn to think, speak, and absorb the other language. This is how I felt during my 13 weeks in treatment.

On The Road of Recovery

So, after completing three treatment programs and working with several very assertive and persistent psychotherapists, I was finally convinced that if I didn't let go of my shame about having bulimia, I would die. It took me some time to come to this realization, but it was this slow transition that gave me my life back. I gradually went from being a bulimic named Aimee to a woman named Aimee who has discovered that recovery is really about learning to live with your eating disorder and coping with it along the way. I see my bulimia as if it were a diagnosis for diabetes. When I look at bulimia in this way, it helps me to separate my association of bulimia with weakness and instead associate it with an illness that needs to be kept in check daily, much like diabetes needs to be monitored.

I know that I must be diligent about meal plans. For me, there are certain foods that are deeply associated with bingeing. If I eat them now, I must have a lot of support and I have to portion size. Pizza is an example. I can go to dinner with a friend who knows about my bulimia and we'll split a small pizza and a salad. That works for me because I get my portion size. But if I have a party and there is pizza left over after everyone has left, I'm terrified because there's a good chance I'll binge on it. Bagels are another problem. I cannot handle the typical office bagel breakfast routine because for me, one bagel was never enough; I ate an entire dozen. Being around bagels makes me very anxious. It helps me to set up and control my environment when food is involved—which it so often is in our society—but that isn't always possible.

I also know that I must make sure I don't get too hungry. If I have an emotional or anxiety-producing situation going on, I know it's time for me to get on the phone. My mom is truly my biggest support system. Even though she lives a time zone away, she's always there to help me. If I need some new way to cope, she brainstorms with me. If there's a stressful situation at work, I need to get out and take a deep breath. I don't binge at that moment; I'm very good at handling the problem at hand. But at the end of the day, instead of unwinding with a hot bath or a book, I tend to immediately go to food. Evenings are still a big problem for me. So I call my mom and I'll tell her what I'm having for dinner, and then I text-message her later. This is my accountability to myself. Being accountable is very important. As long as no one knew about my eating disorder, I could continue to get away with it. As long as everyone around me knows, it's much harder. I can still find ways, but it's not as easy. I associate comfort with food. Instead of unwinding with a hot bath or a book, I have a tendency to turn to food.

Lessons Learned and Applied

There will always be times when I will get anxious about food or a stressful situation and I may binge and purge. But fortunately, I've learned much through the different treatment programs I voluntarily attended and from the therapists and other people whom I met along the way who were suffering with mental health illnesses and addictions. Each of them gave me tools that I still use daily to stay in recovery. My recovery isn't perfect; in fact, it's still a challenge every single day. Sometimes when my emotional stress level is too intense, I binge and purge. But rather than see such episodes as a failure or a character defect, I see them as bumps on the road of recovery. Every day I'm learning to love who I am and recognizing my skills, strengths, weaknesses, and gifts. I've learned to break down problems and anxiety to manageable levels and how to set realistic goals that prepare me for success, not failure. I've also come to appreciate my feelings and to embrace the ones that make me unique.

I challenge the voice of self-criticism that still persists in my head, but I am far enough along in my recovery to recognize that to give in to that voice is a catalyst for a downward spiral to a very dark, lonely place. For many years I tried to fight bulimia by criticizing myself about not being able to "fix" it; that all I needed was will power. Now I manage my disease by accepting it. I honor my feelings by carefully monitoring my food choices and by creating balance in my life on every level, including my career and my personal, social, spiritual, and relationship goals. And I find tremendous satisfaction in helping other bulimics turn their lives around.

For me, there are many tools I draw upon to help me whenever I get anxious. Sometimes one works on one occasion but not on another. Prayer and meditation are very critical for me. If I'm running late in the morning and I don't take the time to slow down and pray and meditate, I feel like I don't manage things well during the day. So prayer and meditation are on the top of my "to do" list every day. For others it may be yoga, reading affirmations every day, deep breathing exercises, guided visualization, tai chi, journaling, writing poetry, painting—whatever works and is healthy is right for that person.

The Dream Revisited

As you can see, there's no fairy tale ending, no resounding "ta-dah!" moment. I thought there would be a sharp contrast between living with an eating disorder and then living without it. It was going to be glorious. But now I know—and I am repeating myself, but this is important—that recovery is really about learning to live with your eating disorder and coping with it along the way. There will always be times when I get anxious about something in my life, and if I'm unable to deal with it and my coping mechanisms aren't kicking in, I may binge and purge. But I've also learned that there are many things that I can do to help myself. As long as I do my best to set myself up for success, my life will go well.

Living and coping with bulimia in recovery is not the same for everyone. In the support groups I run, I see women ages 15 to the late forties. I believe the younger people look up to me. For them, sometimes the bingeing and purging is a dieting mechanism, but often when we begin to talk about it in group, they learn that there are other things going on in their lives—conflicts with their mothers, apprehensions about sex, anxiety about school—that are associated with their bulimia. I have also found that the younger bulimics who have gone through treatment are literally free of the disease. They will probably never binge and purge again. These young women do not have a long history of bulimia, and for them the bingeing and purging was not deeply ingrained as a coping mechanism. Once they realize that their behaviors are about feelings and they get treatment, their eating disorder goes away.

But for the older bulimics, it can be a different story. The longer someone has lived with the disease and allowed the bingeing and purging to become deeply entrenched as a coping mechanism, the harder it is to shake. Harder, but certainly not impossible. Some of these women say they know what their triggers are, but they don't want to look at the underlying reasons for their behavior. They're not willing to give up being thin. But the interesting thing about bulimia is that the longer people binge and purge, the more they disrupt their metabolism. Once they start to eat again, people often lose weight. In my experience it isn't always possible to convince a long-time bulimic of this possibility, however.

A Few Words from "The Mouth"

Unlike most bulimics, I was able to dodge the often devastating damage that could have happened to my teeth, although in the long run, this seeming "advantage" was a disadvantage: if I had suffered damage to my teeth and smile, I probably would have sought help sooner. Yet I learned nearly at the beginning of my bulimia that rinsing my mouth out with a baking soda and water solution after I purged would greatly reduce the harm the stomach acids could cause to my teeth and mucous membranes. Of course, this meant that I had to carry baking soda with me everywhere and at all times, and it added another step I had to take after purging, which meant a greater chance of being caught. So while using the baking soda saved my teeth, I may have saved years of my life if I had had a more compelling reason to seek treatment sooner and/or with more vigor.

Take-Home Messages

That's my story . . . for now. It's a work in progress, and I hope I can help others along my journey. I know that everyone I talk to, everyone who asks me about bulimia or who needs an ear to listen to their story also helps me in my recovery. As for take-home messages, I hope readers find something in my tale that is beneficial. To sum up a few thoughts:

- If you are a bulimic, please get professional help now. You are not your disease; bulimia is a symptom of something deeper, and there are many people and tools to help you. This book is a good place to start.
- If you have a loved one who has bulimia and you want to help her, the best thing you can do is love her, listen to her, and be patient. Let the bulimic know that it's not her job to figure out the reason(s) why she is bingeing and purging, but it **is** her responsibility to reach out and get help and to keep fighting. Tell her you will support her in her decisions, and encourage her to be patient and gentle with herself.
- If you are in recovery, take personal responsibility and make sure you have enough emotional and/or spiritual support. For most recovering bulimics, especially those who suffered with the active disease for many years, every day is a challenge to stay in recovery. Staying on the road is much easier if you arm yourself with many different coping and support mechanisms.
- During recovery, if (when) you slip and have a bingeing and purging episode, don't let it get you down. Reach out to someone or use another coping mechanism to help you get through it. There is always help somewhere: a family member, friend, spiritual guide, stress reduction techniques, support groups, online chats, and hotlines. You have the power to move beyond the bulimia.
- Whether you're a bulimic or know someone who is, remember: It's not about food; it's about feelings.

MAKING UP FOR LOST TIME

Over and over again, people with bulimia talk about how they "lost time" and can't remember or recall many things that were happening in their life when they were actively bulimic. One reason for this lapse in memory is that bulimics often go into a trance-like state when they binge. Because they spend so much time worrying about how and when they can acquire the vast amounts of food on which they binge, then making sure they have safe places and time to binge and purge, they often miss out on much in life. Teenage girls tell how they missed going out with friends or passed up school events because of their bingeing and purging. Some women report how they missed their children's school plays and athletic events and how they feel guilty about "not being there" for their children. Others say they frequently cancelled social events or just didn't show up, that they avoided their friends, begged out of family gatherings, jeopardized their jobs, and become increasingly isolated.

Once these people were in recovery, they learned how to re-enter their world and to restore and rebuild damaged relationships. Counselors, support groups, and family therapists can be helpful in restoring such relationships. It's important for both parties in the relationship to be patient with each other and to practice good communication skills (which can be facilitated by a counselor or therapist if need be) for the relationship to recover. The relationship that blooms from such work can be even fuller and more satisfying than the one the individuals shared before, because now they have shared and weathered strong feelings and come to respect them in each other.

Twenty-seven-year-old Vanessa, whose full story is in chapter 9, had severe bulimia for seven years before starting on the road to recovery. She says that when you begin recovery, you get what she calls "recovery guilt." "You've lost time," she says, "and you've hurt people, missed opportunities and time that you can't get back. So you have a sense of mourning. I've often wondered, 'where did my twenties go'? I was so involved with my eating disorder and the routine of getting up, eating, throwing up, going to work, eating, throwing up, and on and on. That's all I remember, being so structured, and I don't remember a lot of the good things. But once you accept that loss, it's like a spark that rekindles something inside you, and you say you're never going to let that happen again. Now I want to catch up, to participate in life." And in chapter 9 you can read about how she's doing just that.

HOW TO HELP YOUR LOVED ONE IN RECOVERY

If you are the parent or another significant person in the life of a recovering bulimic, there are some things you can do to help him or her through the healing process. Also remember that there are groups and community services that can be helpful as well, so you and your loved one have many means of support during this journey.

Guidelines for Parents and Other Loved Ones of Recovering Bulimics

- Be aware that your attitudes and behaviors about food and weight have a great impact on the bulimic, so keep them positive. For example, keep nutritious foods in the house and help ensure that all household members eat three balanced meals a day. If you need help in planning healthy meals, seek the help of a registered dietician or nutritionist. Such an expert was likely available as part of your loved one's inpatient or outpatient treatment program; you could return to that individual or look for another (see Appendix for resources).
- Encourage family members to eat meals together whenever possible.
- Make mealtimes positive experiences; keep conversations light and do not focus on what foods the recovering bulimic may or may not be eating
- Relapses can and do happen, and the best thing you can do if an episode occurs is to be supportive: offer to listen, reserve judgment, and continue to encourage positive thoughts (see "What about Relapse?" below).
- Encourage the recovering bulimic to share in the shopping and preparation of meals and make them enjoyable experiences. These activities help promote a healthy attitude about food and eating.
- Participate in family therapy. Perhaps you and your loved one attended family therapy sessions previously, but now that he or

she has "graduated" from inpatient and/or outpatient treatment, you may think family therapy is no longer necessary. Wrong! Family therapy is a great resource tool that should be pulled out of the toolbox and used whenever you feel it can be helpful.

- Set reasonable goals. This task is usually best facilitated by a counselor or therapist, because it is easy for bulimics and their loved ones to expect changes to occur quickly and/or for people to be come disappointed if progress seems to stall or the bulimic has occasional bingeing and purging episodes. For example, a recovering bulimic could wake up in the morning and say, "I'm never going to binge and purge again." That sounds ambitious, and if something causes her an unusual amount of emotional stress and she has a bulimic episode, she may view the episode as proof that she is a failure, and that she's never going to get better. However, if she wakes up each day and says "I'm going to try my very best to not binge and purge today and to turn to my coping techniques if I feel an overwhelming urge to do so," then she has set a reasonable goal—she is viewing her progress one day at a time, and calling upon techniques that have worked for her in the past.

- Remember that bulimia is not about food. Therefore, if the recovering bulimic still has occasional bingeing and purging episodes but is showing progress in other areas, such as expressing her feelings more openly, feeling less irritable, making fewer negative comments about herself or her weight, engaging in reasonable exercise (if it was unreasonable before), or going to support group meetings, these are all signs that recovery is moving forward.

What About Relapse?

As I mentioned in the beginning of this chapter, recovery is a work in progress, and so it has ups and downs. Occasional episodes of bingeing and purging can and likely will still occur, especially during the early part of the recovery process. Such episodes don't usually signal a relapse and a return to full-blown bulimia. Rather they are typically isolated incidents and part of recovery. They also can be great lessons, as Ursula explains.

"Whenever I slip and have a binge and purge episode, I look back at it and see what I can learn from it," says this twenty-eight-year-old clothing store assistant manager. "I look for what triggered the episode, what coping mechanisms I tried, and then try to figure out what didn't work so I hopefully won't repeat it. Sometimes I also talk to my counselor about it, and we can work it out together. It's important for me to realize that occasionally bingeing and purging isn't the end of the world; that it's just a mistake, and that I have lots of tools I can use to help prevent them."

Because the possibility of relapse is always a concern, bulimics are strongly encouraged to arm themselves with relapse prevention techniques. Such techniques are typically taught during inpatient and outpatient programs, and are reinforced in therapy sessions and support groups (see chapter 9). In fact, support groups, including Twelve-Step programs, are excellent sources of such tools, as are various other methods, which are discussed in depth in chapter 9.

The important thing to remember about occasional binge and purge episodes during recovery is that they are **not** signs of failure. If your loved one is having occasional bulimic episodes and is avoiding her therapist or support groups because she is embarrassed and feels like she is a failure and has "blown it," it's important for you to listen to her concerns and to reassure her that isolated episodes are part of the recovery process.

BOTTOM LINE

Recovery from bulimia is a highly personal journey, as has been demonstrated in Aimee's story in this chapter, yet there is a kinship among the travelers and among the family and friends who are often an integral part of the recovery process. The encouraging news about recovery, as Aimee has noted, is that there are many support techniques and groups that can help you and your loved ones along the way. In the next chapter, I talk about some of those support approaches.

CHAPTER 9

THE RECOVERY CHEST

One of the most positive things about recovery from bulimia and other eating disorders is the great number of resources that are available to help people through the process. In chapter 5 you read about the first line of defense when it comes to treating bulimia, which includes different treatment options and various types of psychotherapy. But there are even more resources that recovering bulimics and their families can access, therapies and activities that can not only complement any of the first line of defense therapies, but perhaps more important, be a part of the second phase of recovery—the work in progress that we talked about in the last chapter. This part of recovery can be full of supportive opportunities so you or your loved one will always have something or someone to turn to when there's a chance of sliding back into disordered eating behaviors or when a helping hand or words of encouragement would be appreciated.

I encourage everyone to take advantage of as many supportive opportunities as possible. This chapter looks at some of those resources and discusses how they may help you and how you can include them as part of your recovery program.

OPENING THE RECOVERY CHEST

I feel very strongly that the key to recovery is accountability and personal responsibility. So before people with bulimia open the "recovery chest," they must hold themselves accountable and accept personal responsibility for the choices they make and the consequences of those choices if they want to recover fully. Without embracing these concepts, the chances of relapse are extremely high.

Let me quickly emphasize that I am **not** talking about blame or guilt or judgment. On the contrary: being accountable and accepting personal responsibility are very positive and empowering steps that facilitate recovery. I've seen it happen again and again.

This makes good sense if you stop and think about it, especially when we remember that bulimia is not about food, but about emotions and feelings. People with bulimia can blame all their problems—troubles with relationships, job dissatisfaction, an inability to get ahead financially, feelings of inadequacy—on their eating disorder. That is, they believe the bulimia releases them from being accountable for their life because the eating disorder is beyond their control.

Until bulimics are willing to take ownership of their lives and admit that they have made some poor decisions or choices—and it's important to note here that **everyone** makes less-than-desirable choices during their lives, not just bulimics—it is not possible for them to recover from bulimia. Accepting responsibility is not about blame or judgments; it's about accepting the fact that the bulimic behaviors are learned coping mechanisms and as such, they can be changed and replaced with healthy coping mechanisms. The key here is recognizing that **the choice is theirs to make; they have the power to change**. (See box, "Ask Yourself: Am I Being Accountable?")

Ask Yourself: Am I Being Accountable?

- Am I surrounding myself with people who support me?
- Do I ask for help when I need it?
- Am I being honest with myself?
- Am I being honest with the people who support me?
- Am I willing to try new support techniques?
- Do I take the necessary steps to keep myself safe?
- Am I doing the best I can?
- Do I express my true feelings?
- Do I honestly consider the advice offered by those who support me in my recovery?

Once bulimics take back ownership of their eating disorder, they can take the steps and make the healthy choices that are part of the recovery process. Irene, a thirty-year-old respiratory therapist put it this way. "One day it just clicked for me: I realized I was **not** my eating disorder, that it did not define me, although up to that point I had been allowing it to define me. No, bulimia was something I could shed like an old, heavy coat. I was a woman who was wearing a coat called bulimia, and it was up to me to take it off. No one could do it for me. I needed to be accountable and take personal responsibility for my bulimia. Once I realized that, my future suddenly looked a lot brighter, and I was ready to ask for the help I needed to begin recovery."

Again and again I see that those patients who take personal responsibility are the ones who recover from this devastating disease. With the help of professionals, loved ones, and various support mechanisms; these men and women are shedding the coat of bulimia. It's important that they are patient with themselves, that they face their lives without piling on blame, guilt, or shame, so they can learn to make better, healthier choices in their lives.

I am reminded of Nanette. When she was getting ready to complete her six-week outpatient program for bulimia recovery, she took a careful look at her recovery and some choices she needed to make. She considered what the near future held for her and realized she wanted more support. She also realized that she was responsible for finding that support. "Everyone was great during my inpatient stay and then during the outpatient program,'" she said. "I felt safe, and I always had someone to turn to when I needed help. Now I'm about ready to leave the outpatient program, and I think I'm ready to fly solo most of the time, but I'd like a little safety net. I live alone, and my family isn't nearby, so I'm working on establishing a network of support, and the people at the outpatient program are helping me do that."

Nanette is on the right track: recovery from bulimia and other eating disorders is best achieved if you surround yourself with easily accessible support systems. Many people feel apprehensive or a bit "lost" once they complete formal or structured treatment programs and are "back in real life," as Nanette calls it. "Even though I am largely on my own when I'm going to the outpatient program three nights a week, those sessions feel like a lifeboat to me. I think ending them is going to feel like I'm jumping out of the lifeboat, and I want to have a life preserver to grab on to so I can hold myself up."

Fortunately, there are many life preservers for you and your loved one to grab onto. Let's look at some of them and see how they may be able to help you or a loved one through the recovery process.

Support Groups

First I want to clear up any confusion about support groups versus therapy groups, as many people think they are the same, and they are not. Therapy groups are usually run by professional therapists, counselors, or other health experts—people who have experience with eating disorders. They run for a specified period of time; and they are held for a specified group of people, such as those in a residential treatment facility or those registered with an intensive outpatient program for bulimia.

Support groups are generally open to anyone who wants to attend, and people can attend as many or as few sessions as they wish. The goal of a support group is to serve as a focus point where people get together so they can offer each other mutual support, tips, and information. Generally, support groups are run or monitored by people who have some experience with eating disorders, but they are not necessarily professionals. An excellent example is the support group run by Aimee, the recovering bulimic you met in chapter 8 who runs several community support groups for people with bulimia and other eating disorders. Twelve-Step groups are another example of support groups, which I discuss below. (See the Appendix for a list of resources for finding a support group near you.)

Twelve-Step Groups. Although I mentioned twelve-step groups in chapter 6 on initiating treatment, these forms of support are more often used during the ongoing recovery stage. The popular Twelve-step programs, such as Eating Disorders Anonymous (EDA) and Overeaters Anonymous (OA), are based on twelve ideas that participants in the program can use to guide them in their recovery process. Twelve-step groups are usually spiritually based and have a tradition of using "sponsors"—a fellow twelve-stepper who acts as a mentor for a fellow twelve-stepper, offering emotional and spiritual support for that person during his or her recovery process.

Twelve-Step programs typically meet one or more times a week, depending on the need in a particular community. Meetings are free and open to anyone who has bulimia or another eating disorder. Individuals share their experiences, fears, hopes, and ideas with each other so they can solve their common problems and help others in their recovery. According to EDA, "recovery means living without obsessing on food, weight and body image . . . . Recovery means gaining or regaining the power to see our options, to make careful choices in our lives . . . [and] rebuilding trust with ourselves."

Some groups welcome the parents and/or significant others of those with eating disorders, while other locations have specific twelve-step groups who offer support to these individuals. Seventeen-year-old Courtney was glad to see that there was a twelve-step group for the parents and family members of people with eating disorders offered in her town. "It took some of the pressure off of me to explain things," she says. "Even though my relationship with my parents is much better now than it was before I went into treatment, there are still times when I find it hard to explain how I feel. Now I go to my group and they go to theirs, and then we share. It's a big help."

Other Self-Help Groups. Besides Twelve-Step groups, some hospitals, clinics, and organizations sponsor self-help groups that bulimics can attend either free of charge or for a small fee (see the Appendix for a list of resources). The National Association of Anorexia Nervosa and Associated Disorders (ANAD), for example, has nearly 400 groups across the United States and in 18 foreign countries. These local self-help groups offer people with eating disorders and their families a place to support each other. The groups are lead by individuals who have recovered from an eating disorder, eating disorder specialists, or health-care professionals.

According to the results of a recent survey conducted by ANAD, 27 percent of group participants were bulimic, 32 percent were anorexic, 8 percent were compulsive eaters, and 33 percent were a combination of these disorders. Fifty-six percent of the attendees were female, 44 percent male. Ninety-three percent said they would recommend their groups to other people who have eating disorders, and 97 percent the groups were important or somewhat helpful in their recovery process.

How do you know if a certain self-help group is right for you? Here are a few questions you can ask to help you decide. You will need to attend several sessions in order to get a fair sampling so you can answer these questions.

- Are most of the people in the group also receiving treatment from professionals and/or completed treatment with an inpatient and/or outpatient program?
- What is the main goal of the group's discussions: do they focus on providing relevant information by bringing in expert speakers or discussing the latest research on eating disorders or nutrition? Do they disseminate nutritional information?
- Does the group discourage "quick-fix" or faddish ideas about recovery?
- Do the members of the group seem to be improving or seem dedicated to working toward a healthier lifestyle?
- Do the members appear to respect and support each other?
- Does the group's facilitator make you feel accepted and welcome?
- Does the group's facilitator encourage members to seek professional help?
- Does the group promote the idea that maintaining an ideal body weight is a healthy approach?
- Does the group avoid discussions on how to diet, lose weight, purge, use laxatives, or other destructive behaviors?

To help you make your decision, talk to as many of the group members individually as you can and ask them how they like the group, what kind of support they get from the group, and similar questions. If you are satisfied with their answers, and you answer, "yes" to all or nearly all of the questions above, then the group may be beneficial.

Online Support Groups

Technology has brought therapy to our fingertips, and online support groups for bulimics is one of the innovations. Live chat rooms can provide recovering bulimics and others with eating disorders with instant feedback when they feel they need someone to talk to or they want to reach out but they are unable or unwilling to seek live help.

"I attend a self-help group here in town," says twenty-five-year-old Karlyn, who is recovering from 10 years of bulimia. "But at three in the morning, when I can't sleep and I get anxious, I can log on to my computer, go to a chat room, and share my thoughts with others who understand. Online support is a nice option for me."

"Sometimes I just don't want to face anyone," says nineteen-year-old Ryan. "So I go to a chat room, and then I feel better. Many times just chatting with others like me gives me the courage to go out."

Several reputable organizations and websites offer carefully monitored chat rooms and online support for bulimics and others with eating disorders. See the Appendix for a list of these support tools and how to access them.

Spiritual Guidance

The terms "spiritual guidance" and "spiritual therapy," or just the word "spiritual" for that matter, have highly personal meanings for each individual. For some, meditation, yoga, and tai chi—which are discussed elsewhere in this chapter—fall into the category of spiritual therapy, as they have a spiritual component to them. "The thing that attracted me to yoga and meditation was its spiritual component," says Brad, a thirty-one-year-old bulimic who has been in recovery for several years. "The sense of spiritual oneness that I get when I practice yoga, either alone or with others, is very healing. There's a real sense of community and universality."

Others associate "spiritual" with their priest, rabbi, or pastor, or with a teacher from their mosque or temple; basically, anyone with whom you share similar philosophical, moral, and/or ethical interests.

Many bulimics and others with eating disorders who are in recovery find they derive great strength, hope, and comfort from participating in spiritual gatherings, reading inspirational materials, and talking with others who share their beliefs. Indeed, one of the strengths of the Twelve-Step movement, which is spiritually based, is the sense of community that it fosters. Quite a few of the eating disorder centers and programs in the United States are spiritually based or have a spiritual therapy program.

Evelyn is glad she sought spiritual guidance during the early days of her recovery from eight years of bulimia and anorexia. "It was right after I finished my outpatient program," she says, "and I knew I was still vulnerable. Neither my inpatient or outpatient programs had been spiritually based, but there were hints of spirituality throughout treatment, now I was interested in learning more. But I had never been religious and wasn't attracted to anything too structured, so I started reading about different spiritual practices, different religions and belief systems, and I found a common thread among them all: love, peace, kindness. I started attending different services, different groups, and different ceremonies. And it was all very exciting and comforting for me. I know this newfound spiritual life is helping me cope with some of the emotional issues that remain from my bulimic and anorexic days."

Breathing Therapy

It may be hard to believe that something as simple as breathing can have great healing powers, but both research and the experiences of millions of people prove that it does. However, I am talking about *healthy* breathing, not the shallow breathing that comes from the chest and engages only a small fraction of your lung capacity. The vast majority of adults shallow breathe, a type of breathing learned as a response to psychosocial stress. When you learn to breathe from the diaphragm, tension and stress are reduced.

When you breathe in, you take in oxygen, and with each exhalation you release carbon dioxide, a toxic waste. With shallow breathing, you not only don't get the optimal amount of oxygen, you also don't release the maximum amount of carbon dioxide. Sleep disorders, heart disease, fatigue, and headache are just a few of the conditions associated with shallow breathing. Shallow breathing also affects your state of mind, causing you to feel tense, confused, or excited. Proper breathing has a soothing effect on the brain and the nervous system, which helps restore emotional and mental well-being, as well as improves body awareness.

That's where yogic breathing comes in. Yogic breathing is the science of breath control and consists of various breathing techniques that are designed to help you reach and maintain health and to balance the body, mind, and spirit as one. This form of breathing is known as "pranayama": "prana" means life energy; "yama" means discipline or control; thus pranayama means control of the life energy, or breath control.

Pranayama is a form of deep, systematic breathing that delivers energizing oxygen to the body's tissues and in the process improves both physical and mental health. It is used by people who practice yoga to help them prepare for meditation, which I also discuss in this chapter, as well as a means to relax, revitalize the body, and facilitate yoga practice. There are many different types of pranayama, and they can be learned from books or from yoga instructors. One of the more popular forms, called dirgha pranayama, is explained here in the accompanying box.

Dirgha pranayama is one of the simplest forms of deep breathing. It uses diaphragmatic or belly breathing, which maximizes oxygen intake and carbon dioxide release, relaxing the body and mind in the process.

Dirgha Pranayama

1. Sit in a comfortable position with your spine erect, or lie down on your back.
2. Take several long, slow, deep breaths through your nostrils.
3. Each time you inhale, send the air into your lower lungs and allow your belly to expand and fill with air. As you exhale, allow your belly to deflate and relax. Repeat several times.
4. Take a deep breath and send the air into your lower lungs and into your mid-chest, allowing your rib cage to expand outward to the sides. Exhale slowly and repeat the cycle several times.
5. Take a deep breath and this time send the air into your lower lungs, mid-chest and upper chest. Exhale and repeat the cycle several times.
6. Continue with step 5 for several minutes or as long as you are comfortable.

Deep breathing has many advantages: it can be done anywhere, it doesn't require any props, it's free, and it works. I encourage you to try one or more deep breathing techniques and make them a part of your life. See Suggested Readings for some excellent books on yoga and yogic breathing. Once you learn healthy breathing techniques, they will be helpful should you decide to try another beneficial therapy, meditation.

Meditation

Meditation, according to Joan Borysenko, PhD, a well-known author and an expert in the field of mind/body medicine, can be defined as any activity that allows you to keep your attention pleasantly focused and calm in the present. Although there are dozens of different meditation methods, all of them have one thing in common: they all focus on quieting the mind by allowing you to direct all your concentration to one healing factor, be it a sound, image, or your breath. The idea is that when you concentrate fully on one healing element, you are filled with tranquility and calm, and stress and anxiety dissipate.

In today's hectic society, taking time to meditate may seem like a luxury or something that's impossible to do, but it is time well spent and worth investigating. With daily practice, even just 10 or 15 minutes a day, the benefits can be quite impressive. Meditation practices have been scientifically studied in people who have had a wide variety of medical problems, from cancer to chronic pain to migraine to eating disorders, and positive results are the rule rather than the exception.

In a study of women with binge eating disorder, for example, 18 women attended seven group sessions on meditation and also participated in daily meditation practice for a period of six weeks. By the end of the study period, the number of binges per week had declined from 4.02 to 1.57, and the percentage of large binges had declined from 70.3% to 18.11%. The women also reported an increase in control over their eating and mindfulness and a decline in depression and anxiety.

One of the more popular types of meditation is breath meditation. Instructions on how to do breath meditation are in the accompanying box. This meditation form is easy to learn, and like all meditation, it is best to do it daily to reap the most benefit.

BREATH MEDITATION

To begin, set aside about 15 to 20 minutes in a place where you won't be disturbed. Find a comfortable position that allows you to keep your spine relatively straight, whether you are sitting, lying down, or resting in a recliner. Your clothing and jewelry should be nondistracting as well, so loosen anything that is tight or irritating.

Once you are comfortable, focus all your attention on your breathing. You may want to close your eyes, but some bulimics say they feel too vulnerable if they close their eyes when meditating, so it's alright to keep them open or to look down, which keeps the eyes half opened.

- Notice how your breath moves in and out of your nose, your chest, and your abdomen. Let your breath flow naturally; don't try to change your breathing in any way.
- Remained focused on your breathing. If your mind wanders or other thoughts creep in, gently bring your focus back to your breathing. Even the most expert meditators find that their mind wanders on occasion, so don't become anxious over this.
- After several minutes of focusing on your breath in your nose, chest, and/or abdomen, shift your attention to the area just below your navel. As you breathe in and exhale, notice how that area feels. If you don't feel anything, that's okay too. Some people feel a slight motion or tightness; others feel a heaviness. If you don't feel anything, that's okay too; just be aware of the area.
- Now shift your focus to your abdomen and concentrate on how your breath feels when it reaches that area. Allow yourself to remain focused on that area for a minute or two.
- Shift your focus again, this time to your chest, and notice how your breath feels when it reaches that area. Again, focus for a minute or two.

- Move on to other areas of the body, including your throat, shoulders, toes, thighs, hands, and arms, allowing yourself to note how your breath feels in each of these areas.
- Once you have finished concentrating on specific areas, note how your breath feels as it reaches into every cell of your body. Focus for a minute or two on the entire body experience of breathing.
- When you are ready, shift your attention back to your surroundings, take a deep breath, and exhale slowly. You are ready to face the day!

Guided Imagery

If you can daydream, you can likely enjoy visualization and guided imagery. Both of these therapeutic tools have helped countless numbers of people cope with a wide variety of medical conditions, including bulimia and other eating disorders. Visualization is a general term used to describe the use of different visual techniques to help relieve stress and tension and to learn how to cope with different medical issues. When people practice visualization, they enter a state of calm and relaxation and then focus their attention on an image or two in their mind's eye. Guided imagery takes this idea a step further: rather than one or two images, participants take a mental journey through many images, creating their own "movie" or script with a specific goal in mind. For bulimics, that script may include a story line that helps them resist the urge to binge or to feel more comfortable with their body.

Although there are few published scientific studies of guided imagery in people with eating disorders, guided imagery has proven successful in many other medical conditions, including heart conditions, cancer, respiratory disease, depression, and chronic pain. In one of the few studies among bulimics, researchers conducted a six-week clinical randomized controlled trial in which 50 bulimics received either individual guided imagery therapy or no therapy. At the end of the study, treated patients had a 74 percent reduction in bingeing and a 73 percent reduction in vomiting when compared with controls. The treated patients also showed improvement in their comfort level with themselves and their feelings about their body.

The types of images and stories that people create during guided imagery are personal; everyone has images, situations, or scenes that have special meaning for them. You can learn guided imagery on your own from books or tapes, or you can find a practitioner (usually a psychologist, psychiatrist, masters level counselor, or licensed social worker) who can help you become familiar and comfortable with how guided imagery can work for you. Guided imagery exercises can be purchased on tapes and CDs, or you can record your own from a script you find in a book or one your create on your own. If you work with a professional, you may go through two or three sessions (about 30 to 60 minutes each) to help you learn the process. Once you are comfortable with how it works, you can do it at home, where your sessions can be as short or long as you are useful to you. Many patients find that 10 to 15 minutes is the average.

Although there are many different imagery exercises you can use, one of the most popular involves taking a journey to a safe or sacred place (see sample exercise in accompanying box). This could be a deserted beach, the tree house you had as a child, a mountain cabin, or a special chapel. Once you have an imagery exercise that helps you feel calm and relaxed, you can practice it whenever you feel you need it. Some people find that after a while, they can visualize just a few key scenes from their exercise without having to go through the entire guided imagery exercise and get the sense of peace and calm that they need. This "instant" result can come with practice.

Are you skeptical about the power of guided imagery? Consider this: picture someone running their nails down a blackboard. Did a chill just go up your spine? That's because the area of your brain that processes images, the visual cortex, works along with the autonomic nervous system, which controls involuntary functions such as responses to stress. Researchers have mapped this response using a sophisticated imaging technique called positron emission tomography (PET) and shown that the cerebral cortex is equally activated whether you actually experience an event or if you just envision it in your mind.

Safe Place Exercise

You can use this script as a guide to create your own personal guided imagery exercise. Ask a friend or family member to tape it for your so you can use it in your sessions. Whoever tapes it should speak slowly and clearly and pause 5 to 7 seconds every time parentheses like these () appear. The entire exercise should take about 15 minutes, but you can shorten or lengthen it as you wish.

You are about to embark on a journey to a safe place () a place where you can feel relaxed, more in control (). No one can hurt you in your safe place () . . . even if you feel pain or sadness or fear, you will soon feel more relaxed and less fearful, less sad (). Allow yourself to experience the images from your mind's eye () they are part of your safe place.

Let's begin by making yourself comfortable. Close your eyes and take several slow, deep breaths, letting each one out slowly (). Focus on your breathing; picture the air moving into your lungs and out into the space around you (). Notice that you feel more and more relaxed every time you exhale () . . . with every breath you are in more and more control and more and more relaxed ()

Continue to focus on your breathing as I describe some images to you. Allow each of the images to float into your mind's eye as you continue to breathe slowly and deeply () Imagine you are in a special place that is full of peace and joy () . . . that place could be a sandy beach, a meadow full of flowers, a wooded mountaintop, the fort you built as a child, a small island in the middle of a lake, the banks of a gently flowing stream, your grandmother's kitchen filled with the smells of apple pie (). It can be any place where you feel safe and at peace () . . . it can be a place you've been before or a place you've always wanted to go () It can even be an imaginary place, somewhere on another planet or in a different solar system . . . No one else needs to know what the place is because it is all yours () It is the place you can return to any time you feel afraid or lonely or anxious, because you know you will be safe and comfortable there ().

Experience the place you have chosen. Use all of your senses to become intimately aware of your special place () . . . its smells (), its colors (), its sounds (), its textures . . . Focus on the smells () . . . embrace them and breathe them into every cell in your body () . . . become familiar with them (). Focus on the colors () . . . let them wash over you and become one with the colors (). Are they dull? Are they vibrant? Do they pulsate? ()

Focus on the sounds (). Identify each one—a voice, a bird, the wind, running water—whatever the sounds are, let them enter your consciousness (). Focus on the textures () . . . reach out your hand and experience the safe things in your environment—perhaps its water, or moss, or polished wood, or a favorite pet. Experience each texture and enjoy it as part of your safe place.

Look around you and take in the entire view of your safe place () . . . enjoy every sound, texture, smell, and color (). Perhaps you want to create a special bubble around your safe place, to make it even more special and safe from the outside world () . . . your very own inner sanctuary where you can go and explore your emotions and thoughts and understand them () . . . a place that is peaceful and beautiful and calm and always there for you, whenever you need it ().

You can return to your safe place any time . . . simply close your eyes and envision yourself there (). It will always be there for you; no one can take it away from you (). It's there for you when you feel angry or frightened () . . . you can visit it when you want to heal or when you want to feel more in control () . . . It will always be there to comfort you.

You may stay in your safe place as long as you wish () . . . When you are ready to leave, begin to count backwards from ten to one, focusing on your breathing as you do () . . . leaving behind your tension and fears and moving forward with the peace and calm you gathered from your safe place.

Tai Chi

Tai chi is an ancient Chinese practice designed to exercise the body, mind, and spirit and to enhance the flow of energy, or chi (qi), throughout the body in a healing, calming motion. In Chinese medicine, illness and disease are believed to be caused by an imbalance or blockage in the flow of chi. The practice of tai chi can help balance the flow of chi to eliminate illness and maintain health.

Although it has its roots in martial arts, tai chi movements are not aggressive and are based on shifting body weight while moving slowing and gracefully with controlled movements. It has been practiced in China for more than six hundred years, and has recently been increasing in popularity in the United States. According to a Sporting Goods Manufacturers Association study released in 2005, tai chi, along with yoga is the fastest growing exercise among Americans.

Melissa was not aware she was among that growing trend when she decided to go to her first tai chi class after a friend told her about it. Melissa had been attending a support group as part of her recovery process, but she wanted something more. She didn't know if tai chi would be it, but she said she would give it a try.

"I didn't even know what tai chi was," she said, "but my friend made it sound so wonderful I just had to try it." And now she's hooked. "When I practice tai chi, I feel light, like poetry in motion," she says. "I feel good about my body and how it moves. Tai chi relieves any anxiety or sadness I may feel at the time. It helps me stay balanced, and I don't think about bingeing and purging nearly as much. I still go to the support group, but I get something very special from tai chi."

So far, there are no published scientific studies of the effectiveness of tai chi for people with bulimia or other eating disorders. However, tai chi is practiced by millions of people, and countless anecdotal reports reveal that it helps build self-esteem, restores physical, emotional, and mental balance, and enhances a sense of control. Regular practice of tai chi helps quiet the mind and relieve stress, depression, and tension. Since bulimia sufferers can benefit from all of these advantages of tai chi, it seems a natural fit, as many people have found.

Tai chi can be learned from books and videos, but it is best appreciated when done in a class with others and with an instructor who can explain and show you the many nuances of this graceful exercise. Because of its great popularity, it is increasingly easy to find tai chi classes, often offered by community and senior centers as well as private enterprises. See the appendix and the Suggested Reading List for more information.

Yoga

Yoga has a long tradition of helping restore physical and emotional imbalances, and so it is especially suitable for people with bulimia. Scientific research as well as countless anecdotal reports show that yoga helps relieve depression, anxiety, fears, and anger; it also promotes confidence, inner strength, self-esteem, and self-acceptance. Regular yoga practice also helps build strength, balance, and energy, and promotes a positive body image.

According to the principles of yoga, eating disorders are considered to be a dysfunction of the first chakra (a chakra is an energy center; there are seven in the body), which is located at the base of the spine. The first chakra represents the element earth and is associated with survival instinct and our connection to the body and the earth. To balance this chakra, you can practice poses that focus on the base of the spine.

It's beyond the scope of this book to teach you how to do yoga postures, but I list some excellent resources in the Appendix and Suggested Reading List to help you get started. Yoga can be learned from books and videos, but it is recommended that you attend at least a few yoga classes so you can get some one-on-one instruction and gain a better appreciation of what the poses look like and how to breathe properly (more on that below). If you can find a yoga instructor who has worked with people who have eating disorders, all the better; he or she should be familiar with the poses that can be most helpful for your recovery.

Yoga is about more than just poses, however; it is also about calming the mind and achieving inner peace in conjunction with the physical postures. These goals can be realized by learning how to focus your attention on your breathing and your internal sensations rather than on things in your external environment. Both pranayama (yogic breathing exercises; see elsewhere in this chapter) and meditation help calm the mind and body and restore balance to the body as it recovers. While yogic breathing can be especially helpful in reducing tension and anxiety, meditation can help promote a sense of control over one's thoughts and banish the "negative talk" that is so characteristic of bulimia and other eating disorders.

The bottom line is that regular practice of yoga—preferably every day, even if only for 15 or 20 minutes—can promote and maintain self-awareness, self-confidence, and self-acceptance, all of which can enhance the recovery process and your life or that of your loved one.

Energy Healing

The definition of "energy healing" varies, as do the types of therapies that are included in this category, but basically energy healing is any method that addresses the subtle energy that controls the physical body. Several therapies fall into the category of "energy healing," including acupuncture, polarity therapy, touch therapy, reiki, reflexology, and aromatherapy. Although there is no scientific proof that any of these techniques are beneficial for people with bulimia or other eating disorders, these techniques have been shown to be helpful in many other disorders and, in a few cases, are readily accepted by some mainstream doctors and hospitals as part of their treatment programs. In addition, there are many anecdotal reports and in some cases, centuries of use by millions of people, all testimony that these energy healing methods provide relief from stress, anxiety, and depression, as well as help improve self-esteem, body image, and self-confidence.

In my own practice, my team places aromatherapy candles at strategic points throughout the practice to foster calm and tranquility, and the feedback from patients is overwhelmingly positive from virtually all the women and a solid majority of the men. In survey after survey, patients say it is one of the features they most appreciate about the practice. The result is astounding. Indeed, the level of relaxation for both patients and staff is very noticeable.

I will leave it up to you and your loved ones to explore further any of the energy healing techniques that I've mentioned. See the Appendix and Suggested Reading List for sources of information on these therapies.

Therapeutic Massage

Therapeutic massage can be a great way to relieve stress and regain an appreciation of the physical body. "Getting my first massage was both scary and wonderful," says Darrah, a thirty-eight-year-old insurance claims agent who struggled with bulimia and anorexia for more than 20 years. "My therapist was very patient and had worked with people with eating disorders before, so she knew I was apprehensive. But she put me at ease, and even though I was still somewhat tense the first time, I still felt really good after the session. I now get a massage once a month, and each time I feel better about my body, which is really amazing because I've struggle with body image my entire life."

The success of massage therapy in bulimics has been shown in research as well. In a study of 48 adolescent women with bulimia who were also part of a bulimia treatment program, half were assigned to receive massage therapy for five weeks while the other half did not receive massage. All of the women in the massage group improved immediately—they were less depressed and less anxious after their massage sessions, and they scored better on the Eating Disorder Inventory, a measure of psychological and behavioral characteristics in eating disorders. The women in the control group did not improve. Similar research has been done with women who were anorexic, and the results were also positive among the treated patients.

Because you or your loved one may feel apprehensive or self-conscious about getting a massage, it may be best to look for a massage therapist who is familiar with clients who have an eating disorder. To help you find such an expert, talk to your psychotherapist or the therapeutic staff at an eating disorder clinic and ask if they can refer you to someone, or check the resources listed in the Appendix.

Feldenkrais Method

A type of movement education and therapy called Feldenkrais Method, developed by Moshe Feldenkrais in the 1940s, has proved to be very effective in helping people with bulimia and other eating disorders to understand and appreciate their body and feel better about themselves. Feldenkrais conducted in-depth research into the relationship between how the body moves and what we think, feel, and learn. His studies convinced him that how we move is intimately connected with our self-image and that movement plays a critical role in how the nervous system is associated with our sense of self. The goal of Feldenkrais practitioners is to show students how to experience the interrelationship between how they move with how they think, feel, and sense the world around them.

Bulimics and people with other eating disorders so often feel disconnected from their bodies and their feelings, but Feldenkrais can help them reconnect in a safe, relaxing, and fun way. Feldenkrais movements are taught in 30- to 60-minute sessions over a period of weeks to months, depending on how much you want to learn. Gentle movements are used that help realign the skeleton and open up the nervous system. In the process, flexibility, range of motion, coordination, and movement improve. Students often report that they gain new self-awareness, self-esteem, and self-control after participating in Feldenkrais sessions.

Researchers in Germany wanted to document the therapeutic effects of the Feldenkrais Method and so conducted a controlled study of thirty patients with eating disorders: fifteen participated in nine hours of Feldenkrais lessons and fifteen did not participate. The patients who had the Feldenkrais course had increased acceptance of their own body, were more self-confident, and had decreased feelings of helplessness.

Art Therapy

Expressing oneself through art has long been known to be therapeutic for people who suffer with any one of many disorders, and this holds true for bulimia as well. The creative process gives people an outlet for their anger and frustrations, fears and sorrows, and helps them resolve emotional conflicts, foster self-awareness, develop social skills, reduce depression and anxiety, and enhance self-esteem.

Several researchers in Austria put this idea to the test when they incorporated art therapy—painting and drawing—into a treatment program for 36 bulimics. The investigators found that the introduction of painting therapy helped the patients improve their eating habits, reduce food cravings, stabilize their self-esteem, and develop a sense of self-responsibility and work on strategies to manage their disorder.

Life Coach

The concept of a life coach has become increasingly popular in recent years, and for some bulimics, the advice such individuals can provide helps them on the road to recovery. A life coach is (or should be) a professional who offers nonjudgmental support and resource tools that will help you achieve your goals, such as finding a unique purpose in your life, identifying your true vocation, changing your lifestyle, or incorporating spirituality into your life.

According to the International Coach Federation, if you are in the market for a professional life coach, follow these guidelines:

- Know your objectives for working with a life coach: what are your goals? What do you want to achieve? What are your expectations?
- Talk to at least three coaches before you hire one. Question each one on his or her experience, skills, qualifications (especially important when dealing with eating disorders), and ask for at least two references
- Evaluate how each of the potential coaches makes you feel; go with your instincts: do you feel comfortable, did you make a connection with the individual?

I am adding another guideline: if possible, talk to someone (preferably someone with an eating disorder) who has used a life coach. Even though you'll be asking for references from any life coaches you interview, this approach adds another layer of information.

Although this field is relatively new and unregulated, there are several formal training and certification programs for life coaches, and you can contact them for referrals and more information (see the Appendix). I recommend you look for a coach who has a background or a degree in psychology or counseling (in fact, many life coaches are psychologists, therapists, or counselors).

BOTTOM LINE

As I've demonstrated in this chapter, there are many complementary and support opportunities for you and your loved one to take advantage for recovery. Please consult the Appendix for contact information about all of the resources I discussed in this chapter. I wish you much success and joy in your recovery process!

CHAPTER 10

QUESTIONS AND ANSWERS

Throughout this book, I hope I have answered many of your questions and concerns about bulimia, how it impacts your dental health, and how to walk the road of recovery. In this chapter I have brought together some frequently asked questions as well as a few that address specific issues, such as how bulimia affects pregnancy and concerns about insurance coverage. Please consult the appendix for a list of resources that address treatment methods, treatment facilities, health-care professionals, and support groups, as well as a suggested readings list.

DENTAL QUESTIONS

Q. I've been bulimic for about four years, and I'm worried about my teeth. If I brush after I vomit, will that help?

Actually, brushing right after vomiting is *very* damaging to your teeth, because the hydrochloric acid and other stomach acids make your tooth enamel more susceptible to breaking down. If you brush after you vomit, you contribute to the breakdown of your teeth rather than help save them. Some bulimics rinse their mouth with a mixture of baking soda and water (about 1 teaspoon of baking soda shaken with four ounces of water) or plain water after vomiting. Both of these actions provide only *minimal* help and will not save your teeth. **The best way to protect and save your teeth is to get professional help with the bulimia.** Once you have your purging under control, a dentist can begin to restore your smile to its original brilliance.

Q. I've been a bulimic for about a year, and I'm beginning to worry about my teeth. How long before the damage starts?

The damage to your teeth from the stomach acids starts the first time you vomit, but you will probably begin to *see* evidence of damage after about two to three years. You may also begin to notice that your teeth are sensitive to heat and cold, and that your gums are tender, swollen, and/or bleed easily. I strongly recommend that you (1) get professional help for your bulimia, (2) talk to your dentist about preventive dental care, and (3) read my chapter on the impact of bulimia on oral health.

Q. I've been bingeing and purging for about two and a half years, and I recently noticed that some of the fillings in my mouth feel strange; they seem to be higher. What's going on?

As bulimia progresses, the enamel on your teeth is eaten away and your gums recede, which causes changes in your mouth, including the fact that fillings can protrude above the teeth's surface. Over time, the fillings will erode and likely fall out. I strongly recommend you get professional help for your bulimia and talk to a dentist now about restoring your teeth and keeping your smile!

Q. I'm in a recovery program for bulimia, and one thing I desperately want to do is to get porcelain veneers, because my teeth look terrible: they are yellow and don't have any enamel on them. Is it too late for me to save my teeth and my smile?

It's not too late to get your smile back, but you may not get it with porcelain veneers. Fortunately, there are other alternatives. It's necessary for you to have your bingeing and purging under control before restorative work begins so it will last. If it's true that your enamel is gone, then porcelain veneers are not suitable for you, because there must be some enamel on the teeth to which the veneers can be cemented. I suggest you get a full evaluation by your dentist and then look at your options, which may include crowns, bridge(s), and/or implants.

Q. Someone told me that there's a special tooth guard I can use to prevent my teeth from being damaged when I purge. Is that true? And where can I get one?

Your dentist can prescribe tooth guards to help protect your teeth during vomiting episodes. Tooth guards are made of plastic and should be placed over your top and bottom teeth before vomiting. While tooth guards provide some protection, they are not foolproof and they do nothing to correct any of the damage that has already been done to your teeth nor protect the other soft tissues or structures in your mouth, including your gums, salivary glands, throat, tongue, or mucous membranes. They also are NOT a substitute for professional treatment for bulimia, but they can help minimize further damage to your teeth.

Q. I've been bulimic for about three years, and recently my teeth have been getting more and more sensitive to heat and cold. What causes it and what can I do?

First, you should see your dentist for a thorough checkup. He or she will likely question you about vomiting, and I strongly urge you to be honest. Now is the time to get help for the bulimia and to begin thinking about restoring your dental health.

Sensitive teeth develop when the enamel coating wears away or the gum below the enamel has receded, exposing the sensitive inner dentin. At the core of dentin is a pulp chamber that contains nerve endings which are surrounded by fluid and which travel through tubules throughout the dentin and end beneath the enamel. Temperature changes cause the fluid to move, and the movement causes pain.

The best way to treat sensitive teeth due to bulimia depends on the extent of the damage. First and foremost, the vomiting needs to stop. At the same time, your dentist can recommend the best treatment approach based on the extent of damage to your teeth. Treatment options include daily use of toothpaste that contains potassium nitrate, found in products made specifically for sensitive teeth; application by your dentist of fluoride gel or desensitizing agents; crowns; bonding; inlays; or root canal.

BULIMIA QUESTIONS

Q. How does bulimia affect the fetus if the mother is an active bulimic? I'm two months pregnant and purge at least once a day.

Women with bulimia who continue to purge during pregnancy place themselves and their baby at risk. Experts recommend that women who have bulimia or other eating disorders try to resolve these issues before they attempt to get pregnant. If, however, you are already pregnant and are an active bulimic, it's critical that you tell your obstetrician about your bulimia, as you may need specialized care during your pregnancy. You should also seek psychiatric and nutritional counseling to help ensure your health and the health of the fetus.

Purging is normally associated with poor nutrition, dehydration, cardiac irregularities, and chemical imbalances, and during pregnancy these health risks are heightened while even more enter the picture, such as the risk of gestational diabetes, severe depression, premature birth, complicated labor, post-partum depression, and nursing difficulties. Risks for the baby include premature birth, low birth weight, respiratory distress, poor development, and feeling difficulties.

Q. What's so bad about laxative use? I've been using laxatives every day for a few months to keep my weight down.

Laxatives are meant for occasional, short-term use; your description of laxative "use" is really misuse and long-term. The risks of long-term laxative misuse are serious. One is an imbalance in electrolytes and minerals (potassium, phosphorus, sodium) that are necessary for proper functioning of the muscles and nerves. An imbalance in these critical substances can result in improper functioning of the heart, lungs, and other vital organs.

Another risk of laxative abuse is dehydration, which may cause blurry vision, fainting, kidney damage, tremors, and weakness. Long-term use can lead to laxative dependency, which means the colon needs increasingly larger amounts of laxatives to produce bowel movements. Excessive laxatives can also damage the colon, causing it to stretch or become infected, or they can lead to irritable bowel syndrome or increase the risk of colon cancer.

Q. My daughter is very athletic (she's on the track team in high school) and recently has become very conscious of her weight. What are some of the warning signs that she may be bulimic?

There are several risk factors for bulimia and other eating disorders among athletic teens. Participation in any sport that emphasizes appearance, weight, and/or individual achievement (e.g., running, gymnastics, diving) is one such indicator, and your daughter is in that group. Also look for signs of low self-esteem, chronic dieting or unusual habits, or pressure from peers or others to be thin. If possible, become familiar with your daughter's coaches and see if they are concerned about your daughter as a whole person or if they focus only on performance and success, expectations that can drive young people to take extreme measures (such as purging to keep weight down) to perform better. Finally, if you believe your daughter has an eating disorder, learn all you can about it and plan an intervention (see chapter 5, "Step 1: Face-to-Face with Bulimia"). The time to get help is NOW.

Q. I'm the mother of two teenage girls, ages seventeen and thirteen. The older one is bulimic. How do I explain this disease to my other daughter and prevent her from following in the footsteps of her older sister?

I am not a therapist, but going to a family therapist would be a tremendous help in this situation. Remember that an eating disorder affects the entire family, and the entire family can be part of the solution. According to Sherman and Thompson in *Bulimia: A Guide for Family & Friends,* "younger siblings may feel unfairly excluded if not informed about, or involved in, treatment; and not telling younger children might give the impression that they are part of the problem." Often younger siblings bring a fresh perspective to the dynamics of the family and the eating disorder. By including your younger daughter in the solution process, you are helping her as well.

Q. Why do bulimics binge on sweets, fatty foods, and other high-calorie foods?

People binge eat for various reasons: because they are depressed; to cope with overwhelming emotions such as anger, fear, or guilt; because they have been severely limiting their food intake. Sweet, salty, fatty foods are typically carbohydrate-rich and are sometimes referred to as "comfort foods." When someone eats large quantities of carbohydrates in a short amount of time, their neurotransmitter (chemicals in the brain; especially serotonin) production is altered, producing a calming effect on the brain.

Q. How much of a role does genetics play in bulimia?

Researchers have found that chemical changes in the brain may at least play part of a role in the cause of bulimia. Professor Walter Kaye, of the University of Pittsburgh, and his colleagues published an article in the *Archives of General Psychiatry* in which they explained that levels of the brain chemical serotonin (a neurotransmitter that helps regulate mood) is altered when bulimics binge and purge. Serotonin levels remain abnormal, even after bulimics recover from the disease, which indicates that abnormal serotonin levels are not just a result of bingeing and purging, but may contribute to the cause of bulimia as well. Many experts believe that serotonin plays a role in bulimia, which is one reason why the selective serotonin reuptake inhibitor drugs, including Prozac, are used to help treat the disorder (see chapter 6).

Q. I'm twenty-three and have type I diabetes. I've been bingeing and purging for about a year. It seems to be a good way for me to control my weight, but I'm beginning to worry that I may be causing myself more harm. What's the story?

It's not certain how many people with diabetes also suffer with bulimia, but experts believe the combination is common. One reason for this situation is that both diabetes and eating disorders require people to pay close attention to their weight, the condition of their body, and their food intake. Some diabetics who are also bulimic wrongfully believe that keeping their weight down by purging actually helps them prevent the complications associated with long-term diabetes, including neuropathy, blindness, kidney disease, and impaired circulation, but the fact is that bulimia places them at a greater risk of complications, as bingeing and purging greatly disrupt their biochemistry. Since both diabetes and bulimia are serious disorders, the combination can prove deadly, and so the first step should be to get help for the bulimia. However, it is also important that the physician responsible for your diabetes care also be involved in your eating disorder treatment.

Q. I've been bulimic for about five years and would like to get some help, but I don't have any insurance, and I can't afford any of the treatment programs because they are too expensive. Does this mean I can't get any treatment?

First let me say that everyone who has an eating disorder and who wants treatment should be able to get it. Even if that treatment does not include inpatient care at an eating disorder facility or an extensive outpatient program, treatment is available on a sliding scale basis at many facilities, and support groups are often free or charge only a minimal fee for participation. So some sort of treatment is available for everyone.

That being said, it's true that eating disorder treatment is very expensive. The National Association of Anorexia Nervosa and Associated Disorders estimates that the average cost of private inpatient treatment is $30,000 or more per month. Even people who have insurance may find that their insurance company has an annual cap on how many days it will pay for in-patient care. For most insurance companies, that time is only 15 to 30 days, even though this length of time is far short of that necessary for adequate treatment.

So what can you do? Although getting an insurance company to pay for treatment for bulimia can be a challenge, it helps to take all the steps you can to better ensure success. First, make sure you have a diagnosis that has been documented by a physician. Then, review your insurance coverage. There are three major types of health insurance policies: indemnity, preferred provider organizations (PPOs), and health maintenance organizations (HMOs). Indemnity insurance policies are usually the most flexible and comprehensive; PPOs rank next in flexibility and usually require a deductible. HMOs offer the least room for negotiation.

Most policies include mental health benefits, but not all cover hospital or residential treatment, and/or outpatient treatment. Read your benefits booklet and speak with someone at the insurance company about your benefits and what is covered. Getting a clear answer can be difficult, especially from HMOs, but be persistent. Ask to speak with a supervisor or higher authority if you cannot get adequate information. During your call, ask the representative to send you a list of providers they will accept.

If it appears that your insurance benefits are not sufficient to cover the treatment your physician has recommended, contact your insurance company and ask about your major medical benefits. If your health insurance is provided by your employer, you can also ask your personnel department to help you. If you have not gotten any satisfaction from these two avenues, call your state insurance commissioner and explain your situation, including your physician's treatment recommendations and the steps you've taken to get treatment. You should document everything you say in a letter to the commissioner. You can continue further if you still don't get results by contacting your state senators and congress people.

You have other options as well. You can contact any of the excellent eating disorder organizations around the country (see Appendix) for more information and recommendations. They can refer you to local self-help groups that prove very helpful for many bulimics who can't access expensive treatment at a facility.

If you have Medicare or Medicaid benefits, the good news is that many hospitals and mental health centers accept these plans. However, not all of these facilities have professionals who are experienced in treating bulimia or other eating disorders and so are usually not helpful. If you have no insurance or financial means to pay for treatment on your own, you can contact community agencies, which sometimes provide treatment at no cost or on a sliding scale. College students who are bulimic may be able to get help at their college or university student health service or counseling center. Another option is to contact the psychiatry department of medical schools, which often have low-free clinics that are staffed by psychiatry residents.

Some patients find help through a clinical trial. Information about ongoing trials related to eating disorders can be found at: the Computer Retrieval of Information on Scientific Projects; the National Eating Disorder Association (*www.nationaleatingdisorders.org*); the clinical trials registry run by the federal government (*www.ClinicalTrials.gov*); and the MetaRegister (*www.controlled-trials.com*).

Finally, private foundations may be of possible help. The organization A Chance to Heal Foundation (*www.achancetoheal.org*), for example, offers financial support to patients who cannot afford to pay for bulimia treatment.

Q. I'm twenty-eight years old and have been bulimic for nearly ten years. I feel like my life is over; I lie to my family, I lie to my friends, and now that my teeth are getting bad, it's getting harder to hide what I'm doing to myself. I have a good job but I'm lonely and scared, and I'm afraid to have an intimate relationship. But I just can't seem to make myself take the leap and get help. I'm thinking maybe I can quit on my own. Does that work? What do you think?

I decided to turn this question over to Vanessa, who struggled with severe bulimia for seven years before she took the leap and who has experience trying to quit "on her own." Today, Vanessa is thirty years old and has been "clean" for four years. In high school, Vanessa was told by a friend that her teachers and peers thought she had the "perfect" life—she was pretty, popular, belonged to a wide variety of clubs and groups, was an excellent athlete, got good grades—but inside Vanessa felt far from perfect. The kidding from her older stepbrothers about her "chubby cheeks" and baby fat when she was only eight years old lingered in her mind and fed her evolving obsession with food, body image, and weight. By the time she was in high school, she had spent years monitoring her body, engaging in excessive exercise, and restricting her diet. During high school she played volleyball year round, and she worked out four to five hours a day.

But the volleyball and long workouts ended when she entered college, and the pounds began to creep on. She joined a sorority, where her house sisters told her she was a "poor reflection on the house." They hinted that she should become bulimic. And, says Vanessa, "I tried it and was hooked." At one point, Vanessa quit bingeing and purging on her own for about six months, but when she returned to the bulimia . . . well, I'll let her tell you her story:

"My bulimia started at that sorority house, and for the next seven years I would combine bingeing and purging, restriction, and overexercise. After I graduated from college, I was bingeing and purging four to five times a day and experiencing tremendous mood swings which got progressively worse. At times I felt suicidal, with intense feelings of hopelessness, helplessness, and not being able to change anything in my life. At the time I was engaged to my high school sweetheart, Troy, who knew about my bulimia. He told some of his professors what I was doing, and they said I should be "locked up" in an intensive treatment program. I was so freaked out by the thought of being locked up that I began to lie to Troy. Eventually we went our separate ways, although I'm glad to say that today we are friends.

After Troy, I got involved with Brian, and I was glad to have someone who didn't know about my bulimia. I decided I'd be better at hiding it so he'd never know. While I was in college fulltime I also worked part time at a clothing store and also coached teen girls' volleyball. The entire time I was coaching I felt like a hypocrite, as I was telling the girls not to worry about their weight, not to take laxatives, that it was who they were inside that counted, not how they looked, yet I was bingeing and purging every day. I didn't want them to experience any of the things that had crushed me.

After I graduated from college with three degrees (art history, general history, and studio art), I moved to Seattle to be with my fiancé, Brian. He worked fulltime and attended school part time, but I was not working. My bulimia was severe, and I was terribly depressed. My birthday is in early February, and I remember I was so tired of being sick and tired, I decided to quit bingeing and purging. I decided I could do it alone.

That lasted about six months. During that time I got a job as an event planner, and as I was planning a very stressful event, I lapsed and I began to binge and purge even more than I had before. I called off my engagement and started to drink heavily, especially at parties, and passed out often. I was twenty-six years old and didn't care if I lived or died. I did crazy things, like running during the hottest part of the day while wrapped in plastic wrap and layers of clothing. On July 17, 2002, I binged and purged, ran six miles in the heat, came home and binged again. But when I tried to throw up, I passed out because I was so dehydrated. When I passed out I hit my head and was knocked out for hours. When I woke up I was uncoordinated and dizzy, and I passed out again. When I woke up the second time, I decided to stay home for a few days and not exercise, eat, or binge and purge. But when I went back to work, I also went back to the bulimia. I knew I needed help, but I didn't know where to find it.

As an event planner, I had to make cold calls, and many of the calls were to doctors. One of those calls was to a Dr. Gregory Jantz. The person who answered the phone transferred me to his voice mail, and the message said something about bulimia. The message frightened me so much that I hung up. When I called back to leave a message, the voice gave a website address. I visited the website, and when I saw all the help the site had to offer, I began to cry. I couldn't believe it. I sent Dr. Jantz an e-mail and asked him to send me some information. He sent me his book, *Help, Hope, and Healing for Eating Disorders.* I started to read it, and it was brutally honest. I felt like someone had crawled into my life, lived it, and wrote about it.

The turning point occurred on August 17, 2002, while I was at a welcome home party for a friend. I was feeling extremely depressed, hating my life, and feeling unloved, when the four-year-old daughter of a dear friend came up to me. I had to kneel down to talk to her, and when I did, she put her little hands on my face and said, "I love you Auntie Nessa."

Those five words changed my life. I knew I wanted to have a little girl in my life, someone to love so much it hurt. That day I gave up restriction, overexercising, and bingeing and purging, and never went back. I contacted Dr. Jantz about one month after that day, told him my history, and said I wanted help. He asked me to attend his seminar and then to go to his center [The Center for Counseling and Health Resources].

On January 17, 2003, I went to the seminar and one month later I began to see a counselor, Tammy. For the next three and half years I went to see Tammy once a week for one hour, and what I learned during those sessions always stayed with me throughout the week. Even though the sessions were hard, and sometimes I was extremely angry or wondered if I was making any progress at all, I couldn't wait to go, because I wanted to be alive, to fix what I had broken.

About one year after starting counseling I began attending a Tuesday night support group, for which I now am a mentor for girls who are in the intensive program at Hope House [part of The Center for Counseling and Health Resources]. At first I hated the group because it was too hard to verbalize what I was feeling. After the first session I told Tammy that I wasn't going back. She recommended I go a few more times, and by the third time I was hooked. I had found people who knew exactly what I was saying; they understood me, and I felt at home. Soon I also began to attend a Thursday night eating disorders group which is facilitated by a physician and is for people who have gone through intensive therapy or counseling.

Today, for the first time, I love the person I am. I'm okay with the things that have happened along the way. I want to help other people make different choices, to save them from the hurt. That's when real recovery kicks in. The greatest reward I could ever have is to share my experiences and story with others and hopefully help those who have the same problem I had for so long.

APPENDIX

Do I Have Bulimia?

This checklist is a guide that can help bulimics and their loved ones assess an individual's behavior and thought processes to determine if he or she is facing the challenge of bulimia or purging disorder. Rate each of your responses as follows: 1 point for never; 2 points for sometimes; 3 points for often.

- I have an uncontrollable urge to eat, even until I feel physically ill.
- I binge—eat large amounts of food within a very short amount of time.
- I make myself vomit to get rid of the food I have eaten.
- I use laxatives and/or diuretics to control my weight.
- I spit out food after I chew it to prevent ingesting it and gaining weight.
- I use exercise to control my weight.
- I use diet pills to control my weight.
- I use enemas to control my weight.
- I use fasting to control my weight.
- I think about food and eating most of every day.
- I eat bread, pastas, and/or cereals whenever I binge.
- I eat sweets (cookies, cakes, candy, ice cream) whenever I binge.
- I eat dairy foods whenever I binge.
- I eat snack foods (popcorn, potato chips) whenever I binge.
- I eat meat, poultry whenever I binge.

- I eat fruits and/or vegetables whenever I binge.
- I feel tired much of the time.
- I have difficulty with memory and/or concentration.
- I have trouble sleeping through the night without waking up.
- I feel sleepy after eating.
- I have cold hands and/or feet.
- I have bloating, indigestion, gastritis, and ulcers.
- I crave sweets.
- I crave breads.
- I crave alcohol.
- I am terrified to gain weight (lose control).
- I feel fat.
- I find it hard to explain how I feel or to explain my emotions.
- I don't like the way I look.
- I must be perfect and do things right the first time.
- I feel lonely and alone.
- I feel ashamed of my bingeing.
- I feel worthless as a person.
- I have tried to commit suicide.
- I feel like I am never good enough.
- I feel like I have not accomplished much in my life.
- I feel like the demands of life are overwhelming.
- I drink a lot of coffee, tea, or diet drinks during the day.
- I am not willing to gain ten pounds in exchange for no more bingeing and/or purging.
- I experience mood swings.
- I feel like bingeing when I get anxious or nervous.
- I get anxious when I can't exercise.
- I get anxious when people tell me to eat or what to eat.
- I hoard food.
- My eating habits interfere with my family and social life.
- I have lied about the amount of food I have eaten.
- I like and anticipate eating alone.
- I enjoy making meals for other people but don't eat much myself.

Adapted from a questionnaire appearing at *http://www.aplaceofhope.com/evaluations.html* and with permission from Gregory L. Jantz, PhD, CED, at The Center for Counseling & Health Resources, Inc.

0-49: It is unlikely you have bulimia or purging disorder.
50-76: You have some characteristics of bulimia or purging disorder. It is recommended that you gather more information and talk with a professional.
77-105: You likely have bulimia or purging disorder and should seek professional help as soon as possible.
106-147: You have a serious condition and need intensive treatment. Speak with a professional as soon as possible.

Getting Help:

Advanced Cosmetic & Laser Dentistry (Dr. Brian McKay)
Seattle, WA 98122
206-720-0600
www.acld.com
www.bulimiaisadentaldisease.org

The Center for Counseling and Health Resources
Edmonds, WA
888-771-5166
www.aplaceofhope.com

Center for Discovery
Various CA Locations
800-760-3934
www.centerfordiscovery.com

Eating Disorder Center of Denver
Denver, CO
866-771-0861
www.edcdenver.com

Center for Change
Orem, Utah
888-224-8250
www.centerforchange.com

Montecatini
Carlsbad, CA
877-762-3753
www.montecatinieatingdisorder.com

Carolina House
Durham, NC
866-690-7240
www.carolinaeatingdisorders.com

Austin Sendero
Granger, TX
866-549-5031
www.autinsendero.com

McCallum Place
St. Louis, MO
800-828-8158
www.mccallumplace.com

Academy for Eating Disorders (AED)
1-847-498-4274
www.aedweb.org

International Association of Eating Disorders Professionals (IAEDP)
1-800-800-8126
www.iaedp.com

National Eating Disorder Association (NEDA)
1-800-931-2237
www.nationaleatingdisorders.org

www.something-fishy.org
Provides an excellent list of treatment facilities and programs

www.caringonline.com
A site for The Center for Counseling & Health Resources, Inc., it is an excellent source of information on treatment centers, eating disorder clinics, online support, and websites.

www.pale-reflections.com
This site lists more than 200 treatment centers or practices in the US

www.eatingdisordertreatment.com
This site has a long list of treatment centers and practitioners who deal with eating disorders

Psychology Today: directory of eating disorder therapists
www.psychologytoday.com

Eating Disorder Referral and Information Center
www.edreferral.com

Bulimia Nervosa Resource Guide for Family and Friends
www.bulimiaguide.org

Eating Disorders Anonymous
www.eatingdisordersanonymous.org

Healthy Place Support Group
www.healthyplace.com

SUGGESTED READING LIST

Food Fight: A Guide to Eating Disorders for Preteens and Their Parents. Author: Janet Bode

Minding the Body, Mending the Mind.
Author: Joan Borysenko.

The Secret Language of Eating Disorders.
Author: Peggy Claude-Pierre.

The Eating Disorder Sourcebook: A Comprehensive Guide to the Causes, Treatment, and Prevention of Eating Disorders.
Author: Carolyn Costin.

Room to Grow: An Appetite for Life.
Author: Tracey Gold

Bulimia: A Guide to Recovery
Authors: Lindsey Hall and Leigh Cohn.

Talking to Eating Disorders
Authors: Jeanne Albronda Heaton Ph.D. and Claudia J. *Strauss*

Anatomy of Anorexia
Author: Steven Levenkron

Life Without Ed
Author: Jenni Schaefer with Tom Rutledge

When Food Is Love
Author: Geneen Roth

Anorexia Nervosa
Authors: Lindsey Hall and Monika Ostroff

Moving Beyond Depression
Author: Gregory L. Jantz, Ph.D.

Healing the Scars of Emotional Abuse
Author: Gregory L. Jantz, Ph.D.

Annual Review of Eating Disorders
Author: Stephen Wonderlich

Biting the Hand that Starves You
Authors: Richard Maisel and David Epston and Ali Borden

Eating With Your Anorexic
Author: Laura Collins

The Beginners Guide to Eating Disorders Recovery
Author: Nancy J. Kolodny

Just a Little To Thin
Authors: Michael Strober and Meg Schneider

Help Your Teenager Beat an Eating Disorder
Authors: James Lock and Daniel Le Grange

Wasted: A Memoir of an Anorexic and Bulimic.
Author: Marya Hornbacher

Hope, Help and Healing for Eating Disroders.
Author: Gregory L. Jantz, Ph.D

Full Catastrophe Living: Using the Wisdom of Your Body and Mind to Face Stress, Pain, and Illness.
Author: Jon Kabat-Zinn

A Systemic Treatment of Bulimia Nervosa.
Author: Carole Kayrooz

Overcoming Bulimia: Your Comprehensive, Step-by-Step Guide to Recovery.
Author: Randi E. McCabe, et. Al.

Sensing the Self: Women's Recovery from Bulimia.
Author: Shelia M. Reindl

Appetite for Life: Inspiring Stories of Recovery from Anorexia, Bulimia, and Compulsive Eating.
Author: Margie Ryerson

A Bright Red Scream: Self-Mutilation and the Language of Pain.
Author: Marilee Strong

Dying to be Thin: Understanding and Defeating Anorexia and Bulimia.
Authors: Marc Zimmer and Ira M. Sacker